EAT 90% PLANTS:

How Mom, a Hollywood Celebrity and Science Led Me
to a Simple Solution for Healing People and the Planet

Dr. Brian Machovina, Ph.D.

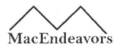

MacEndeavors

For Mom

Let food be thy medicine and medicine be thy food.

– Hippocrates

Contents

Chapter 1: **Introduction**

Covid-19. What will it be remembered for?

How many people it killed? How many lost their jobs? How much money it cost society? I hope at the very top of the list is a clear recognition of what caused it. It wasn't a country. It wasn't a science lab. It wasn't a President.

It was food.

As the closing words of this book were typed out, our global society was still reeling from the pandemic that upended life like no other crisis in our lifetime. Covid-19, the disease caused by the coronavirus known as SARS-CoV-2, has struck the United States especially hard, killing hundreds of thousands of people, driving millions into unemployment, and dramatically changing our perspective on health and the world around us. What is at the center of Covid-19 – the roots of its emergence and the susceptibility of people to the disease – also makes up the heart of this book. Food is at the very center of the pandemic. Covid-19 likely arose from eating wildlife, originating in bats, one tiny example of a global catastrophic over-extraction of wild animals and destruction of their habitat that is dramatically altering our planet to our own peril.[1] People are more likely to experience severe coronavirus illness based on one single factor: if they are obese. It is the most significant risk factor for Covid-19 hospitalization – more than coronary disease, cancer, or even pulmonary disease. With over 40% of American adults obese, the U.S. population was poised to be hit hard.[2] A long list of other expensive, deadly diseases are prevalent due to our increased girth.

The year 2020 is screaming loud and clear that our food choices have profound consequences. First, they affect our own health, which is paramount. We are all selfish beings. We want to live well and live long. We can. Being healthy just feels better. It primarily comes down to what we choose to put in our mouths. Our food. Our drinks. The joy of living together and power of love motivate us the most. We want our loved ones to thrive. We want our communities to prosper. They can. What we eat, serve, and sell to others is the key. We want a clean, vibrant, beautiful world – filled with amazing life-forms – that can be passed on with pride to future generations. We can have that. But we need to make some changes to achieve it. We need to make those changes fast. Fortunately, they are easy.

We are primarily dying due to our diets. The leading medical expenses of our society are driven by our food choices. Radiating out beyond our bodily health is a vast network of interrelated negative effects of our diets on the natural world around us, such as driving most extinctions of plants and animals, massive loss of our life-giving soils, pollution of our waterways, changing of our global climate, and the destruction of the largest and most vital ecosystems on the planet. We are quickly and extensively losing nature and the ecosystem services that support us and humanity's future. We are eating the Earth and leaving a wake of shrinking empty forests and polluted, increasingly desolate, and warming oceans. The financial costs of the environmental effects are enormous and continuing to grow. They will dwarf the direct financial health costs of our diets.

The solution to all these problems is very simple. It is incredibly easy to achieve. It is delicious. It is fun. It is fulfilling. You will be able to walk better, have sex better, and you will feel happier. Your friends and family will thrive. Life will be better! I came to this choice in hindsight, after years of ignorance and mistakes, many journeys and lessons, and inspiring mentors and examples. I am an eternal student eager to learn, question, and change my mind. In my middle age, after a career as an environmentalist and entrepreneur in health and wellness, I dedicated five years to finishing a Ph.D. in Biology. As part of my studies, I intensely examined the three-way intersection of food choice, human health, and global ecosystem health. What I discovered stunned me. I think it will stun you too. It also inspired me because the solutions are simple, elegant, and natural. They are, most importantly, delicious.

I am not pushing you to give up anything in your current diet. You don't have to search for superfoods or buy special powders or pills. A few ingredients you may have never used might pique your interest. You don't have to permanently forgo decadent desserts, snacks, or soda. Celebrating with food makes us human. Most critically, you don't have to stop enjoying meat, eggs, or dairy. The world is not going to turn vegan and you do not have to either. Eating meat is not evil. You are not bad if you do. I eat it. It tastes amazing. All I ask is that you consider making some things more of an occasional treat in your life. Exactly how often you eat these treats is up to you, but this book lays out what I think you should strive for as a goal. A goal to help people and our planet. A goal of 90P: eating 90% plants.

It is my sincere hope that you find this journey and the underlying science enlightening enough to perhaps alter your personal menu to improve your health and that of those around you, help conserve and restore the health of our planet, and better celebrate the pleasure of all food. If we eat 90P, life will thrive. All life.

Chapter 2: **A Mom's Heart**

I hurriedly pedaled my bike down the concrete path, my heart thumping with excitement. I was headed home to Mom to report on the 4th of July party that was developing at our neighborhood park. Woven between my spokes were red, white, and blue paper strips, the colors also wrapped like candy canes around my bike frame and handlebars. Others rippled in the wind along with an American flag. My feet spun around and around fast as my 7-year-old legs could push them, my mouth watering and heart racing from glimpsing the hamburgers, hot dogs, and kielbasa that were sizzling away on the giant grill, the one that came out of the pool house for just this occasion. A few minutes earlier I had poked my head between all the dads discussing and tending the flaming heart of the meal our suburban tribe would soon enjoy. Made from a 55-gallon drum cut in half lengthwise, that big black grill spouted fire and meat-infused smoke, and inhaling the salty and tangy essence of our celebration made my legs pedal with fury toward home. I wanted to tell my mom what I had seen, and return with her to the party. I was going to ride in the parade. Swim. Run races. Play ball. Eat hamburgers. It was going to be the best day of the summer. But on that path home, I came upon a cute girl I had never seen before, her passing smile mesmerizing me like a deer in headlights. My head swiveled back following her as she shrank behind me. I forgot completely about the metal pole that awaited ahead, standing stoic, filled with hardened cement at the end of the path, an impenetrable barrier to cars. As I whispered "who is she?" within my mind, the bike's front tire collided with the cylinder of steel. My body launched, hurtling through the air, and slammed into the concrete on the other side. My face hit the pavement microseconds after my hands tried to break the impact. I rolled and crumpled into a wailing ball of hurt.

I don't remember how I got home, as it was a blur of tears and chaos of frantic voices. What I do remember next was lying on my couch, crying, my mom putting a bag of ice on my face after wiping away the red. My mouth was on fire and my lips throbbed. I had scraped up my hands, elbows, knees, face, lips, and even my gums. My mouth tasted of metallic blood. For me there would be no parade, no swimming, no racing, no baseball. And certainly, no hamburgers. I didn't want to move my swollen lips, let alone chew. I spent the entire day on the couch. My mind wallowed in sadness for missing all the fun and the best meal of the summer. Mom skipped the celebration too, and stayed close by my side. She brought me extra pillows, tucked me under a soft blanket, read me books, and lay by my side stroking my hair. She coaxed me to drink cool drinks through a straw and spooned applesauce into my mouth to squelch the angry hunger in my belly. She had softly transformed screaming pain and chaos into sniffles and snuggly safety. But I dreamed of that grill while wishing I had never seen that girl.

When you think of your mom, what comes to mind? For me, happiness, appreciation, and warm memories turn the corners of my mouth gently upward. You can probably also tell stories of kindness and guidance going back as far as you can remember, a force of caring that could not be matched by anyone else in your life. Memories of tending your injuries, wiping your tears, and easing your fears. Your very earliest memories of life, especially those steeped in compassion, are likely interwoven all throughout your mom. Even those earliest interactions that you can't logically recall are there as a memory imprinted in your very being. Those years she rocked you, swaddled you in softness, and gazed into your eyes may not be recorded as images in your brain, but those moments are remembered by something far more powerful. The supremacy and grace of a mom is that she is the force from which your every newborn cell arose, nurtured with a compassion that spans eons. The deepest and longest bond of your life is that eternal physical and spiritual connection that links you through millennia to the thousands of moms that preceded yours. A mom's love runs the deepest. Through your entire life, from your earliest memories to the last time you felt her touch, I'd bet no one has been there with unending love quite like your mom. Moms nourish us every step of our journey.

I always picture my mom in the kitchen, sitting across the table from me, listening, and sometimes just watching me as I devoured food that she had just prepared. Whenever I walked in the front door, from playing pickup baseball with the kids on my street in elementary school to strolling in from college breaks, she always first asked if I wanted something to eat. She loved feeding my brothers and me, quietly listening to our latest lessons and adventures. If your mom was anything like ours, her cooking was a joyous expression of her love for you. It made her feel as good to feed as it did for us to eat. I have never known a person who gave more unconditional love than my mom. Even when I was at my worst, she was always at her best. Being my mom was not easy. You can ask anyone else in my family. I never colored within the lines. I tore up the paper. At a very young age I rebelled against authority, including her. In elementary school I was a terror. I bonded with other trouble causers. We fed off each other's devious plans and tried to outcompete each other. We glued teachers' desk drawers shut. Put tacks on each other's seats. We purposely clogged the school toilets with toilet paper until they overflowed, finding hilarity in water flooding into the hallway while the teacher gasped in shock. We broke a school window by tossing around a giant roll of brown paper towels, swiped from the janitor's closet, like a football. We tossed it back and forth a few times, until my friend grinned and then launched a Hail Mary far over my head. I watched the paper flutter into a rippling streamer as it crashed through the boy's bathroom window and thumped into the yard two stories down. But one day when the same buddy, sparking a cigarette lighter, suggested setting the school on fire, my mom's stern yet sweet voice whispered in my mind that it was not a wise idea. Thankfully, my path with that compatriot diverged after elementary school. Later in life I learned that he spent many years in prison on a murder conviction for killing a guy with a baseball bat during a drug deal gone bad. He died in his 40s, not as a result of any violent or criminal behavior but because of a heart attack – as odds predict.

I am certain I worried my mom every single day. For nearly the entire fourth grade, I wasn't allowed to eat in the lunchroom with the other kids because I liked starting food fights. The final straw was stomping on a full milk carton, basking in the horror, laughter, and honor that a booming explosion of chocolate milk and scrambling, mortified adults can generate among 10-year-old kids. As cold and isolating as it was to be shunted away from eating with my friends, that experience connected me closer to my mom. No matter how bad I behaved, even after punishing me, she still showered me with love. And her food. Even in deep snow, I had to march 10 minutes from Pine School to my home where my mom had lunch waiting. Little did I know she had a network of friends along the route that would keep an eye out for me, making sure I wasn't distracted and stirring up any mischief along the way, and ringing her on the phone if I was off schedule. When the weather warmed, she would sometimes ride by me on her red bicycle, corralling me more efficiently back to her nourishment and watchful eye.

Of all the lunchtime meals, my favorite was pizza. Lunch was best on a warm sunny day when I could smell the pizza from the backyard as I approached the house across the crinkling green grass. As I slid open the back-porch screen door, the intoxicating aroma made my mouth water in anticipation. The crispy crust, tangy tomato sauce, salty cheese, and spicy pepperoni were spread out in a rectangle on a baking sheet, bubbling with love. This pizza was about as homemade as most Midwestern boys growing up on the edge of suburban sprawl in the 1970s would experience. It was crafted with convenience via the magical, boxed Chef Boyardee Pizza Kit. That meal from a shelf-stable can of sauce and foil-lined bags of preserved cheese and flour – all bundled in a little red, yellow, and green box – was pure nirvana to me.

Every cell in our adult bodies is made up of what once passed through our lips, was ground up by our teeth, then churned and bathed in acid in our stomach, and finally broken down by enzymes and bacteria into carbohydrates, fats, proteins, and other molecules in our intestines to be passed into our blood stream. That pizza and every other bite of food my mom placed on my plate became my bones, muscles, fingernails, hair, and fueled my running stride, the sound of my voice, and the thoughts in my mind. It built me from a dozen pounds to hundreds. Food not only fuels us with calories and the nutrients required to grow and survive, but it binds us with our family, friends, and community. It is the vascular flow of life emanating from the roots of our forefathers. In much of the United States, just like in my childhood home of Ohio, at the heart of that food tradition has long been a hearty helping of meat, eggs, and dairy. Animal-based products. On the vast majority of American plates, one or all of these are served at every single meal in some form. The meals are inviting, mouth-watering, delicious, and are embraced with reverence as All-American, hearty, home-style, and traditional. Between meals, we revel in the ultimate mutualism of free-market business ingenuity and our innate craving for calories: convenience snacks. Infinite combinations of sweet, salt, fat, and flavors in forms that are crunchy, puffy, cracklin', creamy, stretchy, fizzy, and bite-sized have been perfectly engineered by entrepreneurs and corporate giants. This grandiose achievement is displayed nowhere better than in the rainbow of colors and characters in the center aisles of the American supermarket.

Mom proudly called herself a "domestic engineer," managing the chaos of a testosterone-fueled house of a husband, four sons, and no daughters. Cleaning, shopping, cooking, breaking up fights, library trips, doctor's visits, and shuttling among sports schedules filled her days. Her cheeks would flush red and beads of sweat appear on her brow from trips up and down the stairs vacuuming, doing endless laundry, and keeping an eye on the stove, trying to stay one step ahead of her rough-and-tumble boys who were sweaty, smelly, often fighting, and always hungry. At meal time, my mom fed us what most every other family coast to coast enjoyed in the '70s and '80s. Every night, millions of households scooted their chairs in across the linoleum around the kitchen table and feasted on culturally communal recipes, nearly all featuring an animal-based product front and center. Hamburgers. Fried Chicken. Meatballs. Steak. Scrambled eggs and bacon. Ham and cheese sandwiches. Turkey and gravy. Hot dogs. Cereal and milk. Chicken noodle soup. Roast beef. Lamb chops. Barbecue ribs. Meatloaf. Pot roast. Pork chops. BLT. Kielbasa. Beef brisket. Roast chicken. Fish sticks. Pizza. Simply hearing the names made your mouth water. On special nights, you picked up pizza and brought it home. If you were lucky enough to eat out for a birthday or special treat, it may have been a kid-sized burger and fries that came with a toy and a shake, chicken nuggets with a soft-serve ice cream, or if fancy, steak with French fries and a sundae. And for many celebratory dinners out, the food of choice was pizza, but this was the kind that still sizzled and bubbled when it appeared before your eyes on a plastic red-and-white checkered tablecloth decorated with a flickering candle and surrounded by a large room glowing with smiling people.

A side or two consisting of a starch and vegetable accompanied every meal, the starch being the least likely to cause rifts over the offering. Some form of potato – preferably as fries, tater tots, or hash browns followed by au gratin, mashed, or baked – was the most appealing. Rice was a poor runner-up never embraced with much fanfare. The processed boxed version, Rice-a-Roni, with all its flavorful additives, improved greatly upon the original. Veggies were consistently the least appealing, and were there just because Mom said they had to be eaten. They were generally slopped into a bowl from that desolate, solitary confinement of convenience: the tin can. The whine of the electric can opener, the tear of the plastic wrap for the dish cover, and the beeping of the microwave buttons and its subsequent three-minute hum were Pavlov's bells. The standard-bearers of corn, peas and carrots, or green beans were always scooped up with a touch of bland sorrow. The first insult was the mushy texture in your mouth, and then the small pool of grayish canned liquid on your plate threatened to saturate and ruin your crispy fries. The lifeless soggy flavor of canned veggies was contested and palatized with a good dousing of butter, or in my own twist, barbecue sauce. The sugary, smokey tart spice of barbecue sauce made my youth taste better. We all had our food quirks. For every meal I can remember, my little brother Brett only consumed corn as that third pairing behind meat and starch. Of the canned veggies, I will admit it was the most tolerable, and it went great with barbecue sauce. I am certain there is a large cohort of his peers that were silently united across the country in the corn club. A larger club to which my entire family belonged, one which included nearly every American, were those who drank up a full glass of milk with nearly every meal.

When it came to munchies between meals, my mom was a master collector and connoisseur. In our family room, just a step down and around the corner from the kitchen, we had a small closet that we called the snack closet. Though the vacuum cleaner, folding chairs, and a few other occasionally used party-related wares were tucked in there, the majority of the space was dedicated to a wide selection of the exquisitely designed inventions from Nabisco, Kraft, Fritò-Lay, Planters, Kellogg's, and Pepsi that were marketed to Americans in endlessly bright and cheery messages of pleasure through newspapers, magazines, radio, and TV. When I opened the closet door with a friend by my side, their eyes would widen, their tongue unconsciously licked their lips, and a slight swallow of anticipation would roll down their throat. A paradise selection of cheesy, salty, spicy, and sweet wonders awaited us, all lined up in neat colorful boxes that those jingly advertisements primed us to desire. The bounty awaiting may have shifted slightly from week to week, but would regularly feature Cheez-Its, Pringles, Bugles, Combos, Doritos, Fritos, Triscuits, Ritz Crackers, Ruffles, Animal Crackers, Goldfish, Snyder's Pretzels, Twinkies, HoHos, and my favorite, barbecue potato chips. Planters Mixed Nuts were in there too, but only my dad ate those. A single shelf held the cereals in rotation. Fruity Pebbles, Cap'n Crunch, Sugar Smacks, Fruit Loops, and my favorite trifecta of cartoon characters: Count Chocula, BooBerry, and Frankenberry. When buried in scoops of sugar, Cheerios was a tolerable but not very exciting option. On the floor of the closet, lined up neatly on the plaid carpet, were the backup stock of 2-liter bottles of pop, known outside of the Midwest as soda. Pepsi dominated by number, but root beer and Dr. Pepper were my favorite, and a new bottle was always ready to replace the front-runner in the fridge. My mom always had an icy-cold glass of Sprite nearby, nestled on a neatly folded napkin to catch its condensation. But if you wanted something cold, creamy, and sweet, the freezer held a nice selection of ice cream, from Rocky Road to strawberry. Even in the dreary and dirty slush-gray depths of an endless Cleveland winter, ice cream after dinner was still heaven.

The convenience foods and packaging that arose in the 1970s were marketed perfectly to moms just like mine who were looking for relief, a way to free up time to deal with the long list of tasks for the day. My mom beamed with happiness the day my dad brought home a microwave oven – the magic technology scientists came up with to make the lives of domestic engineers everywhere better. In just a few minutes, she could open a can or a box, push a few buttons, and serve her children something warm and delicious. No chopping, mixing, or stirring on the stovetop. It sped up the cycle of nurturing and love. A rainbow of sugary cereals greeted me every day, a staple that made smiles come fast, and morning easier for moms still clearing their heads with coffee. Mom served or packed a lunch whenever I needed it. Leftovers on a white plate, still hot from the microwave, steam pouring out as the disposable plastic wrap was peeled off. Or a brown bag with ham-and-cheese sandwich and a plastic baggy of potato chips. When it was 5 o'clock in the evening, we all had to be home for dinner, and the beeping microwave and warm smells filling the house also filled me with anticipation of quieting the angry growling beast in my belly. Preparing a meal for six people every night was a feat that I never realized at the time was such hard work. As an adult I have learned that cooking for one or two people, just a few times a week, takes a lot of planning to shop, prepare, and time to execute and clean up. No wonder fast food has become such a behemoth. Moms who craft food for their families, filling their homes with mouth-watering aromas, are engineers of love.

However, being immersed in those intoxicating smells but not being able to taste them is a sense memory I will never forget. Truly going hungry in the United States is fortunately not a common experience. Those who have experienced it develop a deep reverence for food that will last a lifetime. To have a stomach shrink and tighten, sour and bitter from days without food, is not an experience anyone wants to endure. Craving food is a force that pulls powerfully, relentlessly on the mind. Cutting out food we love is not a long-term solution. It can drive you crazy, alternating between starvation and gluttony. Anyone who has gone on an elimination diet to shed pounds knows the feeling.

Experiencing the mental anguish, frustration, and anger associated with cutting back on food for extended periods of time was a winter ritual during my youth. In our home, wrestling was the common sports denominator among the four sons. We all wrestled from about the age of 6 until the end of high school, except for Brett, who had a wild fever for wrestling. He even wrestled during the summers. No one else I knew did that. No one. He was crazy enough to take on four more years of the physical and mental beating of wrestling in college, becoming captain of the U.S. Air Force Academy wrestling team. He was a beast. I could probably have taken him in a fight long before high school, but once the wrestling bug really bit him, I knew he could not only beat me in any physical battle, but my two older brothers as well if they joined my side. My entire childhood was filled with wrestling each other at home, and we took great pleasure in grinding our father into the carpet.

I had a love-hate relationship with wrestling. I grew to revel in the camaraderie, the swagger of knowing I was in the toughest sport in high school, and the guidance, tough love, and confidence that only a passionate and demanding coach can offer. But it all came with consistent physical and mental anguish. I always looked forward to the end of the season. High school practices were long and grueling. Our team placed second in the Ohio state championship my senior year. Two to three hours was a typical daily practice session. We always ended practice repeatedly climbing ropes 30 feet to the top of the gymnasium, long after our clothes were soaked and arms rubbery. The walls of the wrestling room would run with streams of sweaty condensation. We all smelled dank and rotten. Practice instilled an ability to be oblivious to suffering that only consistent daily physical challenge can build. We even practiced on Thanksgiving and Christmas mornings. Nearly every winter night for four years, I walked out of practices into the dark, crisp night, inhaling the bitter cold and shuffling to Mom waiting in the warm car, my muscles drained and skin raw. However, what I remember most vividly and unpleasantly about wrestling was being hungry. Very hungry.

Cutting excessive weight for wrestling is no longer allowed, another communal decision made by a society that strives to reduce any discomfort or risk for youth, but it was still widespread in the '80s. You shed pounds in the week before your match, dropping into a weight class where your strength would outmatch the guy normally at that lower weight. However, odds are he was probably also cutting weight. It became an added test of endurance and suffering. Our coach encouraged some of us to cut weight so that our lineup of wrestlers could be structured to have the most talented guys spaced out on varsity. As a 17-year-old senior, I wrestled at 135 pounds. But my body out of season liked being closer to 150. Every week before a match, I would have to typically shed 10 or 12 pounds, sometimes a little more depending on how far off the rails I went eating after my last match. That was when I would, of course, revel in my favorite meal: pepperoni and mushroom pizza from a tiny local Italian pizza shop, Frankie's. That would be followed by a day or two of enjoying normal ravenous three-meal days. And then cutbacks would begin.

About two to three days before a match, the calories were increasingly erased and replaced by the thick, unpleasant concoction known as Ensure, the complete-nutrition drink consumed by elderly people and hospital patients. By 48 hours out, food was often reduced to nothing – no breakfast, no lunch, and no dinner. The snack closet was off limits. As the match closed in, I had to self-ration water to trim more weight. The effort to sweat increased. Running in sweatshirts with a plastic bag, holes torn out for the arms and head, worn as a layer in between, was a staple of weight loss. Wrestling practice was still long and hard, though the day right before a match was a touch lighter. Several times a day, every day, I would hop on a scale and monitor my downward progress. I can still feel the rattling metallic vibration of sliding that scale from under the counter and across the bathroom tile. The whirl of the dial usually bouncing to higher numbers than I'd hoped. This journey was especially unpleasant during the holidays, when tournaments were scheduled. For Thanksgiving and Christmas during high school, I had to skip most of the meals and treats, tortured by Mom's buttery warm aromas in the house. Her food smelled better than ever during the holidays. However, she still would serve up a Thanksgiving plate for me – sometimes just iceberg lettuce with lemon juice and a bowl of popcorn. And maybe a tiny slice of turkey.

Shitting very close to or, divinely, on the day of competition was a blessing that all my fellow weight-losing teammates and I prayed for. If you were lucky enough to have a bowel movement, it was nearly always extremely disappointing in its size. The long bus ride to the opponents' school involved chewing packs of Gator Gum, which is infused with a sharp tang that made saliva flow freely. In the hour before a match, I could fill a 16-ounce plastic bottle with spit, and out went the final pound. Stepping up naked on the scale at weigh-in was the ritual. If successful, that would be rewarded with a warm bowl of beef soup and a bottle of fruit punch flavor Gatorade. The soup-maker role would rotate around the teammates' moms. Brett and I proudly smiled hearing the compliments as our mom's ranked among the very best. She stealthily adapted the purposefully bland recipe that our coach had supplied, slipping in rogue spices. I think she just wanted to spread a little more love to all the grouchy wrestlers. But you couldn't be a glutton and have more than one bowl or drink the entire bottle of that berry sweet liquid. I learned that the hard way, when immediately after a match, I ran out of the gymnasium and threw up crimson mushy meat into a garbage can. My stomach squeezed it out like an angry clenched fist. I felt like shit. Dieting sucks.

Between matches, I spent endless hours dreaming of my mom's food. All kinds of food. An image of dripping pizza sauce was a constant mirage in my mind. I dreamed of drinking it straight from that Chef Boyardee can. However, even a craving for food can be usurped. During the worst stretches of weight loss, I dreamed overwhelmingly of water. In the end, water always trumps food. It is the blood of life. During the final days of intense weight loss, you can discover the true meaning of thirst. The worst morning before a match came when I woke to a tongue drier than anything I had ever experienced before. Its surface had cracked during the night and small bits of dry skin peeled off with the scrape of my fingernail. In my head, it sounded like manila paper rubbing against the roof of my mouth. But I was still overweight and could not risk a drink, or I might end up running in "plastics" to sweat out a half or even a quarter pound right before weigh-ins. That took energy from your match and was just plain misery.

At mid-morning I passed by the kitchen, glancing at the fridge, knowing a full bottle of Gatorade was in there, just waiting for me to crack its cap that evening with a welcoming pop of the vacuum seal. I passed on by and made my way to the basement to wash some laundry. The cool and quiet of the basement was comforting when the irritability of hunger chewed at me. The soothing, gentle sound of the water filling the machine as I opened the lid to put my clothes in was like a siren calling. I was mesmerized by that magical spray of trillions of molecules, two hydrogens and an oxygen, that shot out into the basin. My very survival instincts craved it. Clean. Clear. I stared at the water droplets dancing on the glinting surface as it slowly rose. I crossed my arms and placed my chin on them at the edge of the machine. I gazed into the opening, feeling mist rising up and tickling my face. I just wanted to get closer to that liquid source of life. I leaned in and dipped my head down into the basin. I dropped my mouth wide open and stuck out my crusty tongue, letting that spray of water dance all over it. I closed my eyes and dreamed of waterfalls. It was the most refreshing, beautiful experience I had ever had with water. But I did not drink a drop.

Today, I am a proud member of the clean plate club. Knowing what it is like to deny myself the food I love to the point of anguish and anger, I have a very tough time leaving any uneaten food on my plate. I love food. I understand how others revel in food they love. I love all food. I have tried everything from guinea pig to jellyfish. I consume all the leftovers from dining out that may come home to roost. They often won't survive past breakfast the next day. I jokingly refer to myself as a "scrounge chef" as I root through near-empty fridges and cupboards to find a way to blend strange odds and ends together to craft a meal. I like to clean out nearly everything before shopping for another week's supply. I cherish food and the opportunity to cook in the kitchen for myself and the ones I love. It's a tradition passed on from my mom, but one with an entirely different menu that affects myself and the world around me differently than the food served in her kitchen. Though I love meat, and crave cheese, I lean very heavily on plants. Quinoa with mushrooms and seaweed. Veggie burgers. Curried lentils and brown rice. Tofu scramble. Whole wheat avocado toast. Tempeh chili. Nachos with cashew cheese. Garlicky kale salad. Hot dogs, but made only from plant-based protein. And of course, my favorite: pizza. Homemade, with a sauce cooked on the stovetop, piled with mushrooms, and a hearty sprinkling of nutritional yeast in place of Chef Boyardee's packet of preserved parmesan. I have tried meatless pepperoni, but that stuff fueled enough intestinal gas to fill a blimp. That product needed some more R&D. The mushrooms alone are just fine. My favorite drink is water. It is purely beautiful. I thank wrestling for that. Coffee, wine, and beer are not far behind.

Even with a ravenous appetite and a penchant for eating three meals and snacks in between, of my parents and three brothers, I am the only one who has consistently and effortlessly remained thin. Luckily in my mid-20s, I was exposed to plant-based whole foods – amazingly delicious cuisine – that came to be the base of my diet. It changed my physical trajectory. Though exercise is a supporting factor, my food choices are the primary reason for my lack of body fat. Exercise is fitness, but food is health. As a child, constant physical play, and certainly wrestling, burned up everything I ate and drank. Fat-laden animal products, sodas, and all those processed snacks included. But reduce exercise, add on time measured in years and decades, and the pounds will quickly add up and the arteries thicken. A life of consuming nutrient-deficient processed foods, sodas, and meals dominated by beef, chicken, pork, and dairy will take their toll. Today, over 40% of Americans are obese, and another 30% are overweight. Being overweight is not healthy, nor should we accept it as normal. Obesity is a life-threatening disease that is costing us all billions. The majority of chronic medical conditions, so common they seem inevitable, are caused by one thing: what we choose to put in our mouths.

Animal-based and highly processed convenience foods not only define what we embrace as the norm within our culture, but they literally are what constructed and fueled the vast majority of our bodies. The healthcare costs of this unhealthy American diet are staggering, far more expensive than any other ailment our society faces. It is also a food culture that our corporations have been extremely successful at exporting around the world, generating enormous profits. The health consequences are being exported too. Unfortunately, the typical American diet is a cellular construction and energy source with serious side effects for human beings and the natural world that supports us. Few human actions have caused more environmental damage to our planet than one thing: what we choose to put in our mouths.

The basic meat and dairy core of the American meal, heavily augmented with sugar and fat-laden snacks and beverages, is the order of the day today from sea to shining sea. It is increasingly served up fast and supersized. Unfortunately, it is also increasingly the trend in countries all around the world. As the rest of this book will reveal, the path of the American diet – and the destructive agricultural industry that supports it – can change. We can fuel our lives with delicious foods and thriving ecosystems that will make our lives better.

I wish I could return to an earlier time and share all the knowledge I have gained examining the intersection of food, human health, agriculture, and ecological sustainability. My mom loved to sit at the kitchen table and listen to my every word, even when I was grumpy during wrestling season. If I was disrespectful, many times yelling at my mom with teenage rage, she may have responded momentarily with disappointment and even tears, but always quickly countered with wisdom and love. Like so many moms, she guided me toward goodness. She reveled in hearing all about what I had seen and learned each day. Before I truly understood the nexus of these issues, or had any ability to wisely communicate them to others, it was too late. During my mid-20s and without a care in my mind on a random sunny southern California day, I picked up the phone ringing in my apartment. My older brother somberly told me that Mom had just died.

My mother was obese for decades. She did not exercise. Her diet was the American meat and dairy standard daily for her entire life. She loved soda and snacks. That diet conspired against her and her genes. She suffered from heart and circulatory problems. Prescribed a blood thinner, she died of an aneurism, bleeding out through her nose and mouth in her sleep at the age of 63. My mom was the foundation of comfort and love in my family's life. I cried in my sleep for weeks after losing her, and a profound sadness stayed hidden inside for many years, taking decades to slowly dissipate away. Now I smile with fond memories and gratitude every time I think of her. But I still miss her every single day. I wish I could invite her over, make her a meal, and hear about her day.

Chapter 3: **Blind to Biodiversity**

Do you have a favorite memory in nature? A moment that filled you with awe? I hope so. In our urbanized world, many people rarely experience the primal pleasure of being immersed, undistracted, in the true magnificence of nature. Away from anything man-made. Some people never do. That is very unfortunate. The grandeur of nature has a unique power, like nothing else, to put one's life in perspective, to amaze, to calm, and to refresh the soul. Rolling waves on the open ocean, a shady trail through towering trees, or a tranquil mountain lake. It is perhaps the best way on Earth to get a taste of the amazement that an astronaut feels looking down at the planet. It is what many people seek on vacation – to get away to a secluded beach, a pristine waterfall, or a mountain vista. They amaze. They refresh. They enliven us.

Where I grew up on the western suburban edge of Cleveland, I could roll off on my bike from sunup to sundown with Brett into the fields and woods, beyond the fresh-cut smell of two-by-fours and mortared concrete block skeletons of rising cookie-cutter homes. Beyond those rising sharp-edged geometries were the mystery and nonlinear surprises of nature. Shady, winding trails with flittering birds, slithering snakes, and the whine of mosquitoes. Shimmering ponds brimming with turtles, frogs, and fish. Waving fields with mice, toads, and endless jumping grasshoppers to chase, grab, and watch spit their "tobacco" in our hand – a defensive response of spitting up partially digested plants and enzymes that made us laugh when we sprang it upon an unsuspecting friend. We tromped and waded through many summers. We climbed trees and dipped into cool waters to look, touch, and feel nature. Acorns, bird's eggs, squirrel nests, snapping turtles, praying mantis, garter snakes, box turtles, dragonfly larva, hornet's nests, earthworms, perch, bluegill, catfish, bass, ladybugs, beetles, cicadas, fireflies, hummingbirds, mushrooms, puffballs, and tasty, warm wild strawberries. The pinnacle was coming face to face with a great horned owl, his big yellow eyes blinking slowly, calmly staring into mine. Every new discovery called us to come closer, to look, touch, and smell. The slime of a slug, stink of snake musk, or prick of a fish's spine were our first brushes with threads of life. Brett was always the bravest, first to grab a garter snake and not flinch from the bloody marks it could leave on your arm after a bite. Expeditions a few miles beyond suburbia's boundary felt like we were on the other side of the planet on a safari stalking cobras and tigers. As time and distance would reveal to me, those threads in the temperate ecosystems of Ohio were just a few minor stitches in a living tapestry of life wrapped around our planet. It is a force infinitely diverse, complex, interwoven, stunningly magnificent, and barely understood. It is overwhelmingly underappreciated and undervalued for what it gives freely to us. That young boy had no understanding of biodiversity, ecosystem services, endangered species, nitrate pollution, genetic drift, carbon cycles, or extinction. He was just in awe.

As wide-eyed as those journeys into the wild made a 10-year-old, nothing in my life, before or since, has altered my nature-loving trajectory more than taking my first breath after stepping out of a plane into the heart of the region that quenches the thirst of the entire South American continent. It is the one place with a name that defines wild, mysterious, and biodiverse: the Amazon. My journey there, and perhaps my entire ensuing career, was one of random chance. Though I loved exploring nature as a child, a profoundly uninspiring high school biology teacher veered me away from the "study of life." A wildly entertaining and enlightening physics teacher excited me with space travel, particle colliders, and building contraptions to demonstrate the underlying laws that governed our structures and motion. Solid grades, test scores, and good behavior led to a four-year full-ride ROTC scholarship that took me to the warmth and blessed sunshine at the University of Tampa, where I aspired to be an engineer. Its Moorish architecture, palm trees, sparkling year-round pool, and status as a destination for well-to-do students up and down the east coast, was a gleaming attraction. It was an exclusive, private destination I could never attend without trading years of my future via military service.

However, trailing along with that young man in fatigues was a fondness, one that did not blend well with pursuing a military career, for smoking weed and dabbling in the mind-blowing experiences of LSD and magic mushrooms. I passed the drug test to get into the Army by drinking an entire bottle of vinegar, and abstaining for a couple weeks before peeing into that test cup. But just two weeks into my freshman year, a roommate of mine who had never seen, let alone smelled, the skunky sweetness of cannabis, and was apparently terrified of just the idea of drugs, ratted me out to university administration. Out of Army ROTC I quickly was tossed, and my scholarship was suddenly gone. I was able to finish out my freshman year, thankfully, with support from my parents. They were deeply disappointed but valued me finishing college most. I know they sacrificed to get me through the rest of that year. With the wisdom of hindsight, I am deeply grateful that they supported me in finding my own path, one that they probably had foreseen many times was not destined for straight lines. In the end I only polished my combat boots twice. I quickly found volleyball at the breezy beach and smoking a joint among bikini-clad women far more fun after my classes than crisply marching perfect squares in fatigues under the hot Florida sun. The military life suited Brett, who became a helicopter pilot and eventually a

Colonel in the U.S. Air Force – a career of adventure, discipline, and hard sacrifice.

I kept my grades high, but I also chased getting high. Mushrooms, LSD, and cocaine flowed in freely via my new replacement roommate and friends down the dorm hall. I dropped acid a dozen times, wandering the emerald landscaping, glassy black river, and sleek skyscrapers that edged campus, touching and marveling in the fractal details of palmettos, barnacles, and towering glass and concrete. I bonded with an ever-smiling student down the hall named Matt, son of a wealthy gold dealer from New York. He taught me what an eight-ball of cocaine was and all the creative ways to score one well before his fat allowance came in from home. He took me on adventures to the sketchier parts of downtown to pawn and then repurchase his stereo several times in order to fund all-night revelries he threw. Friends crammed into his dorm room drinking, smoking weed, laughing until we couldn't stand, grinding our teeth and talking cocaine-fast until sunrise. As spring break approached, I had no plans to go anywhere as the $20 my mom mailed me with a loving letter every week was a small sliver of joy that gave me the financial freedom of pizza and beer, certainly not a bag of coke or a vacation. But Matt would not allow that lonely fate for his friend. He offered to help take me somewhere, anywhere we wanted to go. He would have plenty of cash to cover most of a journey for both of us. His family had a home on an island in the Caribbean we could hang at or maybe head to the beach parties of Mexico or Ft. Lauderdale. However, on a random weekday afternoon between classes, we proposed choosing our adventure another way, a gamble that would change my life forever.

Facing each other and propped on our sides on my dorm room floor, we pondered the horizons lying before us. Splayed open wide on the scratchy gray industrial carpet was the great blue and green world. An oversized atlas was opened, our hemisphere covering two pages. Matt deftly rolled a joint, a thick yet tidy one where one end had a girth about twice that of the other – a little bat. Bob Marley, through his sunny melody about those upbeat three little birds, encouraged us onward. Matt gave me the honor of sparking up the fat end with a lighter. I took a drag and passed it on over to my generous friend. We basked in the familiar tradition for a while, listening to the paper and plant crinkle as they glowed orange and creeped slowly toward our lips. We spun the big book around without looking at it and closed our eyes. Each of us stuck out a finger and dropped it down onto the world below. We opened our eyes, our two fingers thankfully landing closest well to the south of us. I really wanted to go somewhere far. With hesitation, then rolling into laughter, we knew this destination would be unique. Nobody goes there. It was wild. And dangerous.

In 1989, Colombia had the highest murder rate in the world.[3] On average, 60 people were killed every day, and less than 1% of cases were solved. At the center of this wave of violence was the Medellin drug cartel and its notorious leader, Pablo Escobar. At the height of his power at that time, his true net worth was unknown but estimated at over $25 billion, making him not only the richest criminal in history, but one of the richest men in the world.[4] The cocaine production and distribution enterprise that Escobar managed was likely the source for our all-night parties on campus. At the time, I knew or cared little about where that white powder came from or the larger effects it was having in the world. For about six months of my life at the risk-taking age of 18, cocaine was a fun and exciting new adventure, but one that is gladly only a distant memory in my past. It runs strongly countercurrent to a healthy life.

In November of 1989, Escobar and the Medellin Cartel were responsible for the single deadliest criminal attack in Colombian history. In an attempt to assassinate presidential candidate Cesar Gaviria Trujillo, the cartel placed a bomb onboard Avianca Flight 203. Moments after taking off, the plane exploded over the town of Soacha, killing all 107 people on board. Eight months before that horrible event, Matt and I boarded a flight to Bogotá, Colombia. We had another set of tickets for the following day that would take us south into the tropical frontier depths of the country. For our spring break, we wanted adventure. We wanted to smoke Colombian weed. We wanted to snort Colombian cocaine. We wanted to journey into the unknown heart of it all. But we wanted to live to tell about it.

Back in the days before computers and artificial intelligence packed planes with maximum efficiency ticket sales and flight schedules, commercial airliners often had many open seats. But this flight was near empty. We were certainly the only two young white American boys onboard that flight from Miami to Bogotá. Our presence must have seemed odd. Halfway through the flight, another man about our age who passed us on the way to the toilet, paused next to us upon his return. After a moment, he plopped down in a seat across the aisle. He nodded and politely inquired about where we were headed. He had a caramel complexion, thick wavy jet-black hair, and spoke English quickly with a sharp accent. He was a funny, friendly guy. He introduced himself as Juan, explaining that he was from Colombia and was attending college in the States. He was headed home to see his family during spring break. When he learned we were on a very non-structured vacation adventure deep into his homeland, he was shocked, and grew very concerned. We did not yet have a hotel booked in Bogotá, any U.S. dollars exchanged for Colombian pesos, and we spoke very sparse Spanish. I had taken just two introductory classes in high school. About all Matt could say was "Hola," with a big smile and a strong, very non-silent emphasis on the "H." Central to the adventure for us was figuring it all out along the way. Luck was smiling on us. Juan appeared as a first, friendly step in figuring it out.

Juan's dad was picking him up at the airport, and he insisted that he would take us to a safe hotel for the evening. He could also help us exchange dollars. It sounded like a good plan to us, but in the back of my mind was a tickle that we might be in the process of being scammed. Just as he said, Juan's dad greeted us, and after a minute of fast banter in Spanish between them that I could barely follow, his father introduced himself. In perfect English he insisted, very politely, that would he help us get settled in the city for the night before we flew out the next day for the Amazon. The wariness in my mind dissipated, as the four of us departed the airport in a very tight compact car, and the excitement of my first vacation in a foreign country unfolded before me. Juan's dad had an easy, calm demeanor, and a smile that mirrored his son's. He explained how he would exchange dollars for pesos with us personally to get a much better rate than a banker would give, but he needed to get cash at an ATM. As I learned in the coming many years of traveling to Latin America, people were always eager to have stable U.S. dollars.

Driving through Bogotá was jolting, chaotic, and edgy with a cacophony of blowing horns, roaring muffler-free tailpipes belching black clouds, and near misses with people darting through traffic. Cars, buses, motorbikes, bicycles, and people dodged one another. My eyes were wide and jolted by the grittiness, the litter, and the shocking level of poverty that was evident along our route. My throat burned from diesel exhaust. Adults and scores of kids with no shoes, clothing soiled to dark sooty gray, and hollow, despondent looks in their eyes were widespread. They gathered in pairs on curbs, walked among the cars at stoplights, and begged for change just beyond my face and the thin glass that separated us. I had seen homeless people during trips to downtown Cleveland as a child and several lived in the park around my campus, but the street people of Bogotá lived a life of emaciation, barefooted-ness, and filth that astounded me. It was exhilarating, humbling, and frightening.

I was in awe to see life so counter to anything I had ever experienced. Juan and his dad paid no attention to those ghosts walking around. I realized the background noise of life in a country like Colombia was nothing like mine. It was raw, gritty, and tough. Juan's dad soon stopped the car on the side of a road in the center of Bogotá, turned around, and told us to lock the doors and stay in the car. He hustled across the sidewalk over to a glass box on the outside of the tall concrete building next to us, an enclosure slightly larger than a phone booth. It contained an ATM, attached to the building's wall. I had never seen an ATM in a glass box before. Juan's dad entered the box and closed the door behind him. Traffic honked and sped by us, and we patiently waited for him to return with a stack of pesos. After a few minutes, I saw him open the glass door again, but he suddenly stopped and looked to his right, and then back at us with a calming pump of his open hand. It was that universal signal to just sit tight.

In a fury of rapid honking, revving engines, and metal scraping, three cars condensed together about 30 yards away from us, screeching to a halt. Two of the cars had forced another up onto the sidewalk, and a group of men erupted out of the two on the street. They were yelling and aiming pistols and submachine guns at the third car. They quickly opened the doors and pulled the men in them out and onto the sidewalk. In a jostling, command-barking struggle, the armed men shoved the others against the same concrete building that held the ATM booth. One man on the wall turned and argued, but was shoved back, gun barrel pointed at his head, others' hands patting him down. There were no police uniforms. The other people out on the streets around us scattered away.

I remember thinking this looked just like a movie, and then felt my heart take off and sweat seep. Matt, Juan, and I were so focused on the action in front of us, we forgot about Juan's dad, until Juan turned to the back seat, yelling at us to follow him. I turned and saw his dad frantically motioning us to the booth. We bolted from the car and four of us squeezed ourselves into that little glass box, the door locked behind us. Juan told us not to worry, as this booth was bulletproof. Just a precaution, he said. But as quickly as it started, the action was over. The men hustled the others at gunpoint and rearranged themselves into the three cars, and they sped off.

We slipped back into our car and took off of in a hustle for the hotel. Juan turned to us and said, "Bienvenidos a Colombia."

From the moment the flight took off the following morning, my face was pressed against the window. The gray squares of urban Bogotá spread out in the valley below, ringed by undulating green peaks. We jostled through turbulent Andean mountain air, rising over mist-shrouded ridgelines. Soon passing below the window were the emerald and olive checkerboards of crops and rolling pastures of humanity's last influence spilling out from Colombia's central valleys. I love the vantage point from a plane. It gives such a grand perspective, a sense of wonder looking down upon humans so small that an individual being can't be seen, just our collective footprints. It makes you feel tiny, yet connected and aware within the enormity of our people and planet. Columns of clouds billowed around. The plane hurtled through, dipping, tipping, and shaking on all the moisture swirling up from Earth. As we rose to over 30,000 feet, the flight smoothed. The clouds broke and scattered. The terrain below had flattened and turned green. An unending green. Green as far as my eyes could see. The surface was unbroken except for the meanders of dark rivers, sunlight glinting off each subsequent sinuous curve as we raced overhead at 500 miles per hour. I got up from my seat and looked out the other side of the near-empty plane. It looked no different. A carpet of tropical forest was spread out as far as I could see, white pillars of puffy clouds rising up like smoke. The jungle passed by far below us. I thought of jaguars, pythons, and dark waters. My heart thumped.

When I stepped out of the jet's door, I was halted. Not by the view, or the sound, or the smell. But by the feel. It felt like sucking in a breath of warm liquid with the flavor of fermenting leaves, fresh-cut grass, and a pond in the woods. Uncomfortable heat. Oppressive heat. It reminded me vaguely of a steam room at the fitness center. Thick, wet, but with a rich earthy heat like I had never felt before. The sun seared my skin and battered my eyes. Sweat dripped down my back within my first few steps down the stairs to the black runway. By the time I reached the short line of taxis under trees on the other side of the one-building airport, massive wet spots were spreading on my shirt. Sweat streamed down my crack and soaked my underwear. The pavement was dark and sizzling from a just-passed rain, and moisture boiled up all around. We had set our spring break destination as far south in Colombia as we could go, into the heart of the Amazon forest. Leticia is a frontier town, a trafficking crossroads between three countries: Peru, Brazil, and the land of Escobar, across which we had just hurtled in air-conditioned comfort that I quickly missed. Leticia's humidity is consistently and relentlessly above 85%. After tossing my backpack into the trunk of the taxi, I looked up toward the sun bearing down on us with a wincing squint. It was my first trip south of the equator. That imaginary line encircling the planet, marking the region that's closest to the sun, was just 300 miles to the north. Along its span thrives the richest, most biodiverse life our planet harbors. But biodiversity was not a concept that my mind had even grasped at that time. The jungle was an edgy backdrop for our journey. Matt and I were after adventure. And drugs. In Leticia, both came quickly.

Within an hour we were sitting on a bench under a giant tree drinking a cold beer and eating our first empanadas, which instantly became the staple of our diet. They reminded me of Hot Pockets, the perfectly cubed pepperoni and cheese-stuffed frozen American treats that were microwaved inside a silvery carboard tube to create a semi-crispy exterior. We discovered empanadas by pointing into a case, choosing something that looked familiar – crispy fried dough that hopefully held happiness. Oh my, did they. These hand-crafted empanadas were the lightest and crunchiest pocket, a tasty turnover made with savory yellow corn dough stuffed with seasoned beef mixed with cooked potatoes. They were perfect for breakfast, lunch, and dinner, and could be taken and eaten anywhere. The two of us must have eaten a hundred during that week. Before we had finished our first one, a young boy appeared next to us. His clothes were soiled and torn. He looked barely a teenager. And hungry. We held out an empanada to him, and he smiled. He grabbed it and devoured it. He spoke to us excitedly, but we understood very little as he chewed, other than a muffled "que rico!" which I remembered from my Spanish I class in high school as the universally important "Delicious!" Our first friend in Leticia quickly became our travel agent, an underworld insider who knew the streets. He recommended what we should visit, areas to avoid, and introduced us to jungle guides he ensured would meet our unique wishes. All he wanted in return was some food. He would eagerly eat anything we gave him. I remembered my parents telling me to clean my plate because there were starving children in the world. They exist. This one was named Carlos.

I clumsily explained to Carlos that we were there to see the jungle, the mighty Amazon River, and, quietly whispering, to do so enjoying what Colombia was famous for – marijuana and cocaine. After more hand waving and rough, fumbling translation among us, Carlos darted off. Fifteen minutes later, he returned with a victorious smile. He unwrapped some crumpled newspaper. In it was a big wad of brown marijuana, overdried, full of seeds, and very poor quality. Back in the States, this would have been called "dirt weed." But it was weed. Then he slipped an oversized matchbox out of his pocket, and slid open the little drawer from its cover. The interior was filled to the rim with a tan powder. It looked very different from the fluffy white powder found in Florida.

"Cocaina?" I asked Carlos.

"Si! Basuco," he smiled back. He pointed to the weed and basuco. "Diez pesos."

Matt touched and tasted the creamy powder with his pinkie, and rubbed it on his gums. He nodded with approval. He handed Carlos a 10-peso coin, which was about 5 U.S. dollars, then another.

"Para ti. For you," I said. "Y los hongos?" I asked.

Carlos started walking away and waved us to follow. He led us through muddy, litter-strewn streets with boney dogs digging in piles of trash, and eventually down to a wide slope descending to the famous waters of the mighty river. At the top of the slope, we paused. The Amazon coursed by, carrying along huge chunks of the forest. Giant logs. Entire trees on their sides, their emerging halves reaching toward the sky with fluffy leaves. Clumps of grass. Rafts of weeds. They all swirled on by in the coffee-and-cream water. The sun relentlessly beat down, and a constant sweat had entirely soaked my white t-shirt. Colorful blue, red, and yellow wooden boats crowded the bank, and people were loading and unloading fruits, palm leaves, plastic jugs, fish, lumber, and baskets. The river, wide and brown, flowed by. It was massive. Intimidating.

Carlos waved us down the slope to a long, skinny wooden boat half covered by a palm thatch roof and mounted with an old outboard motor on the back. A shirtless man in cutoff jean shorts and flip-flops held out his hand for a strong-gripped shake. He bore a foot-long hunting knife hanging on a black leather belt around his waist, but also wore a kind smile under the frayed edge of his woven hat. Matt and I climbed aboard, packing enough plastic water bottles and empanadas, crinkling in plastic bags, to survive a day. We soon watched Carlos and the rusty tin roofs of Leticia slipping into the distance behind us. I dipped my hand into the Amazon, pleasantly surprised by the coolness, and scooped up water and poured it down the back of my head and neck. Matt and I each snorted a bit of the basuco, which was as poor of a quality of cocaine as was the weed Carlos had scored for us. *Basuco* is the word for cocaine paste in Colombia, which is derived from *basura*, the Spanish word for trash. It roughly means "little dirty trash" of cocaine, referring to the crude extract from the coca leaf. Cruising down the Amazon and winding our way into smaller tributaries, we could not have been happier with the raw coca high enjoyed at its source. Inspired, we lit up a harsh, throat-burning joint from Carlos's crumbly brown weed and the rolling papers Matt so prudently packed for our vacation. We laughed at each other, reflecting on traveling all the way to the Colombian Amazon to score the lowest quality drugs money could buy. It seemed a minor inconvenience as the swirling river below us and the forest around us became the powerful force that filled our minds with wonder and awe. With an hours-long drone of the motor, we watched tall, dense walls of green trees and tangles of vines passing by us on both sides, growing closer and shutting out more of the burning sky as the river twisted and narrowed. I nibbled on an empanada, my eyes wide at the jungle drawing in on both sides. The shade of the canopy darkened as we weaved our way deeper into the depths of the forest. My heart thumped.

Suddenly, the sun beat down hot and harsh again. I squinted and pulled my cap down over my face. The forest had abruptly and dramatically opened. It had virtually disappeared. On both sides of the narrow tributary, the trees were all gone. The high river bank was covered in tall thick green grass. Our guide angled the boat toward a muddy V-shaped opening in the bank, revved the throttle for a second, and ran the bow up into the red soil until we were solidly held by shore. Cutting the engine, he hustled past us, grabbed a rope from the bow, hopped onto the bank, and bounded up a slope into the grass. He turned, motioned us to follow, and disappeared into the emerald blades. The mud splatting below my boots was the color of rust and slick like ice. Slipping up that little slope painted my hands and knees. My heart raced with excitement as I finally reached the crest, grabbing at the grass to pull myself up and go from knee to boot to vertical. Matt scrambled up next to me.

"Fuck," was all he could mutter.

Spread out before us for hundreds of acres, was grass. Bright green thick-bladed grass. It was low, undulating, and mottled with clumps reaching knee high. It spread out before us under a burning sunshine that made the skin wince. The whining rhythmic hum of insects filled the air so loudly that it was deafening. On the far side of that enormous grassy field was a dark low wall of trees where the forest edge stood stark and linear. Between us and that sharp edge were scattered hundreds and hundreds of waist-high, crusty-black burnt stumps where giants once stood. Some were the diameter of coffee tables. Contrasting the charcoal skeletons of combusted trees and the vibrant emerald carpet of fresh life were hundreds of white figures. They all stopped and stared at us in unison.

"Mmmmooooooo!" Matt bellowed loudly, then laughed.

Laid out before us was a vibrant green pasture filled with cows, not the fat Midwestern black-and-white cows on a Ben and Jerry's ice cream carton, but skinny, dingey white cows. Their ribs and other bones poked out prominently, giving a cubist topography to their skin. I thought perhaps the tropical heat prevented them from ever getting fat. No doubt it would me as I felt I was sweating out my body weight every hour. As they stared at us, their tails swatted continuously at flies and insects buzzing around. Their ears flapped. One after another, they decided we were no threat, returning to pull and chew at the grass. Our guide waved his arm at the open field rolling into the distance, beckoning us on to our treasure. Matt and I stomped through the grass. Just as the search began, it ended. In seconds I was staring down at a wide, spreading thick paddy of cow shit, about to place my boot into its gooey center. Another waited just a step away. Flies buzzed and snacked on their dark moonscape surface. Matt and I looked at each other and bumped fists. Sprouting from that second pile of shit was the magic we were seeking. *Hongos.*

It seemed every other pile of cow dung bore the white mushrooms with a tan-tipped cap. These were psilocybin-containing mushrooms. Magic mushrooms. There were thousands, probably millions, in all directions around us. Matt reached down and picked one with a cap the diameter of a drink coaster. He grinned ear to ear, pointed at it, and I snapped a photo. He ate it. I selected my own and forced it down with wincing grinds of my molars. As always, they tasted terrible. Like shit. Water and another empanada eased the disgust, but we knew the discomfort would be worth the journey to come. Within an hour, the effects would kick in and take us on a mystical mental journey into the great unknown. I had eaten magic mushrooms before, but I had never picked them. No one I knew had ever eaten them in the depths of the largest tropical forest on the planet. We nodded at each other with victorious pride. The shopping bag that we filled with a couple pounds of fresh-picked fungus could last well beyond spring break.

The experience of cocaine may be difficult to explain to someone who has never snorted a line, but the journey of psychedelics is truly impossible to describe. Psychedelics open a window in the mind that cannot be relayed to others via words, songs, video, or any other form of human communication. You have to experience it to understand it. Your own ego and your past experiences, against which you compare new encounters, dissipates. You look at life, and every detail you encounter, with the wide-eyed wonder of a child. You glimpse into another dimension of consciousness, sensing a closer underlying meaning in life. But you never truly understand it. It is "awe" magnified a million times. Nothing in life's experiences is as magical or mystical. Nothing. It is a mental kaleidoscope of discovery, enhanced perception, and a deeply reflective peek into something larger in our minds and life that cannot be matched. It can be wonderful and healing, but only with the right mindset, setting, and preferably with experienced guidance.[5] I have had experiences filled with terror that I would not wish upon anyone.

The rest of the day and the ensuing week were filled with vibrant, joyful, reflective, and deeply conscience-altering experiences, many made possible by befriending the well-connected and street-savvy Carlos who opened doors to acquaintances that only a street kid could. Gliding through towering forests flooded 20 feet deep with seasonal rains. Fishing for piranhas in oxbow lakes at sunset but struggling for hours in twilight to nervously restart a rickety boat engine. Being visited by pink river dolphins rolling to the surface of inky black water, their breath puffing us with a rainbow of mist. Capybaras, which look like dog-sized guinea pigs, scattering across sand bars dotted with enormous jaguar prints. Lakes filled with lily pads big enough to float a child on, their blood-red lower surface hidden below the water and covered in a carpet of inch-long spines. Visiting smiling indigenous tribes that wore nothing but grass skirts and lived with zero modern amenities. Getting robbed at gunpoint by a border guard whose checkpoint shack was wallpapered with the crudest of centerfolds. Shaking hands with a spider monkey. Feeling the breath of a jaguar on my face. Push starting a derelict taxi while wondering if the driver was about to make a run for it with our backpacks in the trunk. Visiting a well-hidden camp full of very friendly people and seeing bricks of cocaine neatly piled for export. Touring a Colombian naval vessel full of equally friendly people fighting those very same drug traffickers. We were the only gringos the region had seen in a long time, and we were strange baby-faced curiosities. We had little fear of the unknown, and as years would pass, I came to realize how little I understood or appreciated during my first foray into the Amazon. I read next to nothing about it before we journeyed there. I was young, naïve, ignorant, and like so many others on this planet, oblivious to the details of life around me. I was in the middle of the most massive, biodiverse ecosystem on the planet, but I understood zero about it or what it provided for life on Earth. Wisdom takes time. And inspiration.

On the flight back to Miami, Matt pulled out a small handful of mushrooms from a plastic bag in the pocket of his filthy, rusty-red soiled pants. They were some of the last we had from that first day's magnificent harvest. Those mushrooms and the empanadas we devoured, both of which fueled our minds and bodies during our journey into the Amazon, were born from its destruction. That field of deforestation that rolled into the horizon, replaced by grass and beef cattle, came at the expense of destroying countless species of uniquely spectacular plants and animals, some maybe never even discovered by humans. It caused soil loss, took away land critical to survival of indigenous tribes and wildlife, and fostered regional and global climate change. It was my first glimpse into the loss of our planet's great biodiversity and its global regulatory systems that make our lives possible, but at the time, the concepts did not even register in my mind. The starkness of that cleared forest was jarring, but it rewarded me with pleasure. Beef empanadas. Mushrooms. I had never been taught anything about tropical deforestation in high school. There was so much forest all around that overshadowed that scar from which we picked our bounty of shrooms that it seemed insignificant. How my understanding would change.

That first journey into stifling humid, vibrant tropical life, steeped in psychedelic reflection, had planted a desire in my mind to explore more. I was pleasured far more by its nature than its narcotics. Reflecting on that flooded forest that had towered around our boat as we wove among its massive giants would increasingly fill my dreams for years to come. My mind opened and yearned for its secrets. I soon devoured books about jungles, alive with beasts I had not yet seen: anacondas, kingfishers, electric eels, and caimans. Motivation seeds understanding. How little I comprehended while racing across the sky in that aluminum tube back to the United States. However, my mind was already yearning to discover new exotic destinations, high from the adventure of delving deep into an explosion of life. But my immediate attention was on dinner. I ended my first journey into the rainforest by slicing up the last of that magic shit-tasting fungus and mixing it into the gravy topping the beef dish on the tray table in front of me.

Chapter 4: **Profits of Death**

How do you think you will die? Everybody wonders about it at some point. Many of us prefer to never reflect on the possibility. Some people dwell too much on it. Death comes for us all and in many ways, some sudden and unexpected and others diagnosed, battled, and drawn out. Brett and I used to jokingly contemplate about the worst ways to die. Shark attacks. Snake bites. Wasting away with cancer in a hospital bed. I think I settled on dying of thirst in a desert, unable to even lift an arm, watching buzzards softly land around me, hearing them approach to first tear at my eyes while I still barely clung to life. People have died in far worse ways, terrible nightmares everyone wishes to avoid. Death can be cruel and callous.

At the heart of living is avoiding dying, but walking near the edge of death can also be exhilarating. Ask any race car driver, big wave surfer, free climber, sky diver, or mountaineer. The risk of dying can make life exhilarating. I have accompanied Brett on a handful of high-altitude mountain-climbing expeditions. Of the 54 peaks in Colorado higher than 14,000 feet, he has summitted all but one. He sometimes climbed two or three in a single day, and skied solo from the final peak all the way back to his car. I've joined him in the depths of winter when the temperature in our tent pitched above tree line dropped to 30° F below zero at night. On every attempt, I never made it to the summit. Highly susceptible to altitude sickness, partially from living at Miami sea level and flying in for climbs just days later, I always reached a point of pounding headache, nausea, and stomach-emptying vomiting that pummeled me into turning back. The challenge, which included a risk to my survival and climaxed with glorious views, even if not on the peak, drew me back to try again several times. My most memorable and accomplished climb with him was on Pico de Orizaba, also known as Citlaltépetl. It is a stratovolcano, the highest mountain in Mexico and the third highest in North America at 18,491 feet. The upper reaches are capped by a perennial glacier that requires crampons, metal spikes attached to your boots, and ice axes to climb. Most people would use safety ropes to link climbers together in case someone slipped. We went without.

After hours climbing through black rocks and volcanic ash that absorbed the beam of our headlamps, the sun began to rise. We started our trek up the glacier, our spikes biting into the hard ice. We passed over bridges of ice spanning the first of several deep, dark blue crevasses. My brother stopped, turned to me, furrowed his brow, and said sternly, "Don't slip. Don't fall. If you do, you will die."

On those upper reaches, an un-arrested slip could lead to a screaming, rapidly accelerating slide down the rock-hard ice and a freefall deep into one of the crevasses. Worse than broken bones, bloody contusions, or organ damage would be the melting of the ice around you by your body heat, which would refreeze and lock you solidly into place to slowly die, thirsty, shivering, and unable to move. That death could give the buzzards competition. I didn't slip, but the underlying risk made my every step purposeful, focused, and driven. For hours the background of my mind cycled through the people and moments of life that I cherished most. A soul-diving and mind-opening sense of Zen arises when you walk the edge of life, focused on survival. After more than five hours of climbing, I made it to the volcano rim, but I knew climbing the remaining distance to the highest point was just too risky. I had dried Clif Bar vomit splashed up to my knees. Any water I drank quickly came back up with a stomach clenching retch. I had to fight very hard in my own mind to stay focused and alert in the thin air. One of the worst headaches of my life squeezed my skull in a vice. I just wanted to lie down and sleep. But that was not an option. Thankfully, the way down was much easier, sliding slowly on my side and butt in glacial ice that, under the rising sun, had softened the top few inches to the consistency of a snow cone. That glacier, the Jamapa, no longer exists today. Climate change erased it by 2001, only seven years after I crawled upon it — a quick death for an icy realm in a rapidly warming planet.[6] I am by no means an accomplished climber, but I have dabbled enough to taste the draw of the climb, the feel of the edge. Facing death is living life.

For most people, little pleasure comes from flirting with death. At the heart of our very survival mechanism are instincts that help us avoid it. You reel in disgust from the smell of another person who used a toilet before you because the gases released, like hydrogen sulfide, are highly toxic and the offensive odors are a warning sign of potential risks to human health. This is because others' waste can be rife with harmful disease and our instincts know this. A slithering snake can make people leap away in terror, triggered because humans evolved alongside these creatures, many of which are deadly. This fear saved the lives of our ancestors and through many generations, it became innate behavior. However, people are terrified by fear of death from causes that have an extremely low chance of affecting them. The chances of dying from a venomous snakebite in the United States is nearly zero. About six people die from venomous spider bites every year. Eight times as many perish from bee and wasp stings. On average, only one shark bite fatality occurs every year. Only 50 people out of the nation's more than 320 million citizens die from lightning strikes. About 800 people die in bike accidents.[7] Deaths caused by animals, acts of nature, or recreational accidents are extremely rare, but people are highly motivated and encouraged by society to avoid and mitigate many of these low-risk dangers. A shark sighting can close entire beaches. Millions of spiders get squashed and sprayed. Sirens warn of approaching lightning storms. Bike helmets are ubiquitous. However, people put very little attention or effort into avoiding the most likely causes of death and chronic debilitation, and our society has made few concerted efforts to reduce the risk. This is likely because the leading driver of death also generates enormous profits for many interdependent industries, from farming to medicine. Profits trump health.

Take a moment during your day, at any random time, to look at the people around you. Perhaps you will be sitting among your family watching TV, strolling through your office, sipping a coffee in café, or cheering in a stadium packed with tens of thousands of people. Odds are zero percent of those people will die from sharks, spiders, lightning, or bike crashes. However, about one in every four people you see before your eyes will likely die of cardiovascular disease (CVD). You, your family, friends, and all your fellow screaming fans included have about a 24% chance of dying from it.[8] It is the leading cause of death in the entire world. Almost half of the U.S. population suffers from CVD, which includes coronary heart disease, heart failure, stroke, and hypertension. It is driven overwhelmingly and universally by one decision: the food we choose to put in our mouths.

Poor diet quality is responsible for a greater portion of cardiovascular disease-related illness and death than any other risk factor.[9] Adding in diabetes and strokes, which are also driven by this same dietary pattern, adds about another 8% to the odds of death. The final odds predict that about one of every three people you see around you will die from heart disease, stroke, or diabetes, which are deaths ultimately caused by an underlying chronic unhealthy diet. The diet that is killing us is comprised of far too much beef, chicken, pork, fish, eggs, dairy, and highly processed foods laden with sugar and fat and devoid of fiber and nutrients. It fuels obesity and all the associated diseases. And yet we as a nation do very little to address this underlying cause. Selling these products and treating the cascade of debilitating health issues generates profits, and lots of them. Who would want to slow this gravy train of money that would have the practically immediate effect of helping people live healthier, more vibrant, and longer lives? Hopefully you, even if it's just for your own selfishness. I changed my eating habits for that very reason, but also discovered it could have enormous impacts on the entire planet that supports me.

The most likely cause of your death are foods that are marketed and sold to you and your loved ones every day through non-stop advertising, drive-throughs, delivery apps, school lunch laws, government subsidies, and even sponsorships of health-promoting non-profit organizations. The animal product industry generates enormous amounts of income and supports many jobs, and understandably they fight very hard to maintain that stream of income. The size and economic importance of the industry is massive. The meat and poultry industry is the largest segment of U.S. agriculture, accounting for over $1 trillion in total economic output or about 6% of gross domestic product (GDP).[10] The meat and poultry industries are broadly responsible for over 5 million jobs, which is about 3% of all jobs in the U.S. The dairy foods industry directly employs nearly 1 million workers and contributes more than $200 billion to the national economy.[11] In 2019, the U.S. egg industry produced the equivalent of 300 eggs for every U.S. citizen, providing over 100,000 jobs that pay billions in wages and taxes.[12] Together, these animal product production industries are incredibly profitable, powerful, and deeply ingrained in our nation's culture, economy, and government.

The outlets that sell these foods to consumers are equally massive. Setting aside supermarkets, casual, and finer dining, the fast-food industry alone is huge. Its menus are dominated by animal products like burgers, fried chicken, pizza, and milkshakes. Powerful corporations like Yum! Brands Inc., McDonald's Corporation, Burger King Worldwide Inc., Wendy's International Inc, Jack in the Box Inc., Dunkin Brands, Domino's Pizza Inc, Papa John's Pizza, and Dairy Queen are the dominant players with universally recognized brands and powerful legal and lobbying power. Globally, the industry is worth over a half *trillion* dollars.[13] In the United States, revenue was $200 billion in 2015, which is enormous growth compared to the revenue in 1970 of $6 billion. Over 200,000 fast-food restaurants are spread across the United States and it is estimated that 50 million Americans eat at one of them daily. The fast-food industry employs over 4 million people.[14]

Adding to the animal-product-centric foods of these industries are the processed food and beverage industries that create convenience products with long ingredient lists of unpronounceable names. The empty calories, fats, flavorings, additives, sweeteners, and preservatives of convenient foods and beverages tap into the innate biological craving to maximize calorie intake, which evolved many thousands of years ago to help our hunter-gatherer ancestors survive periods of food scarcity. The U.S. packaged food market size was estimated at over $800 billion in 2016, and is steered by market behemoths such as Coca-Cola Co, Nestlé, The Kellogg Company, Conagra Foods, General Mills, and Kraft Foods.[15] Most of these products are made extra delicious with the addition of one key ingredient: sugar. About 80% percent of the 600,000 consumer packaged foods sold in the United States contain added sugar.[16] We are also quenching our thirst with sugar. Sugar-sweetened beverages dominate drink sales, which include regular soda, fruit drinks, sports drinks, energy drinks, sweetened waters, and coffee and tea beverages with added sugars. On any given day, about one half of all Americans drink a sugar-sweetened beverage. All this added sugar adds up. Today, the average American consumes over 125 pounds of added sugar each year.[17] *That is 3/4 of a cup per day!* This consumption drives massive profits and numerous jobs. Soda production in the U.S. has an estimated market size of over $250 billion.[18] At the root of this sweet addiction is the sugar production industry, which is estimated to generate $20 billion a year in economic activity and over 140,000 jobs.[19]

The economic incentive to protect and grow this profit-generating system is at the heart of an epidemic of the "lifestyle diseases" like obesity, cardiovascular diseases, and diabetes that have infiltrated our society to such an extent that they have become normalized and, to some degree, even embraced. We now focus efforts on reducing body shaming instead of reducing promotion of the foods and beverages that are the root cause of obesity and the cascading list of health issues associated with being overweight. We encourage body pride, even if you can't see your own penis because of your belly, which is the case for about one in three of my fellow men.[20] I wouldn't be proud of that. It would tell me that my body is out of balance, that my chances for health problems, need for pharmaceuticals, and an earlier death are greatly magnified. My stamina would be greatly reduced. Love for food has to be tempered first with care for ourselves. Who doesn't want to live a long life? A healthy vibrant life. Eating healthy means being selfish – self focused. Shaming others is not the solution, but encouraging pride in healthier eating and people making efforts to do so is, in my opinion, the best kind of pride to promote.

Calculated from a formula involving height and weight, body mass index (BMI) is a measure of body weight health. According to the CDC,[21] a normal or healthy BMI is below 25. A BMI of 25 to 29.9 is considered overweight. The cutoff for obesity is 30. The average American has a body mass index (BMI) of 29.4. During my travels, I am always curious to ask foreigners what they think of Americans. I was raised to see my country as a leader, a beacon of inspiration. With head-shaking pity, the leading descriptor I hear, especially from Europeans, is usually "fat." We are fat. Very fat. And it is costing us a fortune and killing us. However, many people are making a financial killing off making us fat and keeping us that way. They are in full support of body acceptance and personal choice, promoting their products as a part of a balanced lifestyle. Cigarette companies once employed similar strategies. At the root of our national healthcare problem is money: who makes it at whose expense.

A good example of profits driving poor health options is pizza, a major contributor to the estimated average American intake of over 650 pounds of dairy products per year.[22] I remember my high school lunch line having pizza as an option every day, offered up by the familiar raspy-voiced, unsmiling lunch lady, "Peeeza or pasta?" I always chose pizza, and I still love it. Nothing matches the aroma of a fresh-baked pizza pie or the perfect balance of crunch, tang, fat, and salt. But I have learned to enjoy the version with real dairy-based cheese as a rare treat at most a few times a year. When your diet becomes dominated by plants, your own body gives you an indication of what cheese does. If you eat a diet rich in plants, that is dominated by whole foods, you will notice the effects of just one serving of cheese. The following day, your daily morning ritual of a very smooth, fluffy, and easy-passing poo will be disrupted by a sticky clog in your pipes. Brett and I used to refer to cheese as "butt cement," and for good reason. It's sticky and gooey going in your body and coming out. The constituents of cheese, digested, pass through your intestines and essentially make your blood thick, sticky, and gooey, and slowly help build up plaque on the interior lining of your arteries.

Think of arteriosclerosis, the hardening of your arteries, like a layer of cheese that is laid down slowly layer upon layer, often starting very early in your life. The plaque is made up of very similar groups of molecules as those found in cheese and animal products in general: cholesterol and fatty substances. Your genes also play a role in this artery hardening, but it's the food that fuels it. Eating animal products is the root driver of arteriosclerosis. Like a high-application setting on a paint sprayer, your body may be genetically predisposed to eagerly lay down saturated fats and cholesterol, but if you cut off the supply of paint, or fill the device only on rare occasions, the buildup on the surface is greatly hindered. This coating on your arteries becomes thicker and inhibits flow. Immune cells traveling with the blood mistake these fatty deposits for intruders and attack. This causes chronic inflammation that makes the plaques more likely to swell, rupture, and lodge somewhere like a dam, cutting off blood flow. When this blockage occurs in a vessel supplying the heart muscles, this causes a heart attack.

Over 700,000 people in the U.S. have a heart attack each year, enough to fill seven of our largest football stadiums.[23] About

120,000 of these patients die. If a chunk of this plaque breaks off into your blood stream and travels to your brain, it can become lodged and block blood flow. Stroke victims could fill another eight stadiums, with about 140,000 of them dying. Many studies indicate that eating animal products is also closely linked to developing type 2 diabetes.[24] The number of Americans with diabetes could fill 300 stadiums. The disease prevents your body from using insulin properly, resulting in unusual sugar levels that can build up in the blood. Research suggests that one out of three adults has prediabetes, but nine out of 10 of these people don't even know they have it.[25] Diabetes increases atherosclerosis-related inflammation, and diabetic patients are twice as likely to have a heart attack or stroke.

On any given day, about one in 10 Americans will eat a slice of pizza, generated from an industry that earns about $50 billion in annual revenue.[26] We see advertising for pizza, dripping and with stringy melted cheese, everywhere. It can arrive hot at your door in less than 30 minutes. It waits nearby to satisfy your cravings, frozen in millions of our kitchen freezers. It is a staple of office celebrations, school lunchrooms, and kids' birthday parties. The pizza and dairy industry would like nothing more than for us to consume more of it. And to add extra cheese. Or show your meat lover's pride and top it with pepperoni, sausage, ham, bacon, seasoned pork, and beef. They even came up with the idea of stuffing cheese *inside* the crust. About a decade ago, members of the industry lobbied the U.S. Congress to have pizza essentially count as a vegetable in school lunches, thanks to its smear of tomato paste.[27] Seriously. Only an eighth of a cup of tomato paste, high sodium and added sugar included, spread on a slice of pizza is credited with as much nutritional value as half a cup of vegetables. When I do math, an eighth of a cup is four times smaller than a half a cup. This funny legislative trick enables better profits for pizza manufacturers making a school lunch product that magically magnifies a little smear of sauce into a "serving of vegetables." The joke is on us as nearly one in three of our kids are overweight and one in five are obese, progressively marching through school toward diabetes, hardened arteries, and heart attacks.[28]

I know as well as anyone how amazing eating a slice of pizza can be. It has been my life-long favorite food. It smells and tastes amazing. It just makes you feel great when you eat it, and soon calls you back for more. One reason it is so revered is the cheese. It is addictive, just like a drug. A study published in the U.S. National Library of Medicine examined why certain foods are more addictive than others.[29] Pizza came out on top of the most addictive food list, and it's all about the cheese and its main constituent protein, casein. During digestion, casein releases opiates called casomorphins, which attach to the same brain receptors as heroin and other narcotics. Each bite of cheese produces a tiny hit of dopamine. Dr. Neal Barnard, founder of the Physicians Committee for Responsible Medicine calls cheese "dairy crack."[30] Kicking the cheese and dairy addiction can be very difficult. Vegetarians will eliminate meat products, but often continue consuming dairy. However, the health improvement that comes from eliminating or dramatically reducing dairy intake is reflected simply by body weight. Studies have shown that shifting to a vegan diet leads to more weight loss than a vegetarian diet that includes dairy.[31] Other studies have shown that vegans have significantly lower BMI, overweight, or obesity values than meat eaters, fish eaters, or vegetarians.[32] The benefits to your body and health go way beyond just the weight loss. The basic recommendation from leading experts – the American Heart Association, American College of Cardiology, the USDA, and the Department of Health and Human Services – is that cardiovascular disease is best addressed with a healthy dietary pattern abundant in fruits, vegetables, whole grains, legumes, nuts, and seeds, and that includes small amounts of lean unprocessed protein sources (including poultry and seafood), fat-free or low-fat dairy products, and liquid, non-tropical oils.[9] Remarkably, only two out of every 1,000 U.S. adults has a healthy diet score as defined by the American Heart Association.[33]

I could write volumes worth of information on the health consequences of a diet sparse in plants but dominated by animal and processed food products, but others before me have already done eloquent and exhaustive accounts. They have my deepest respect and gratitude as pioneers, as they have certainly been the target of powerful industries that profit from promoting the opposite. The first book I ever read on the subject was *Mad Cowboy*, by Howard Lyman, a fourth-generation Montana cattle rancher who watched his loved ones suffer and die from the very products their family produced.[34] Becoming vegan, he stood up against the beef and dairy interests that were intertwined with his family's legacy. He bravely faced massive financial and legal power to expose animal-based diets as a primary cause of cancer, heart disease, and obesity in this country. He, along with Oprah Winfrey who declared that the discussion with Lyman on her hit TV show "has just stopped me cold from eating another burger," were sued, alleging more than $10 million in damages, by members of the Texas cattle industry for making false statements about the safety of food. After a six-week trial, Lyman and Oprah won with a unanimous jury decision. I bought the book after attending an impassioned talk by Lyman, who was humble, kind, and caring. That book, and personally diving into and out of 100% veganism over many years, led me to many other great books. An influential one was *The China Study*, by Doctors T. Colin Campbell and Thomas M. Campbell.[35] In it, they examine the link between the consumption of animal products and chronic illnesses such as heart disease, diabetes, breast cancer, prostate cancer, and bowel cancer, based on a 20-year study examining mortality rates from cancer and other chronic diseases on 6,500 people in China. It is one of the largest dietary health studies ever performed.[36] The conclusion is clear that one can escape, reduce, or reverse the development of numerous diseases by eating a predominantly whole-food, vegan diet. Another excellent book, written by their colleague and cardiologist Dr. Caldwell Esselstyn, is *Prevent and Reverse Heart Disease*.[37] In it, he argues for a low-fat, whole-food, plant-based diet that he has since prescribed hundreds of times successfully to dramatically improve people's health. However, an anecdote from one cardiologist using plant-based diets to treat heart disease that has stuck most prominently and durably in my mind was one that helped me see why we continue to have a massive problem with widespread unhealthy diets. From production to treatment, like most issues, it boils down to money.

Dr. Jami Dulaney, through simple dietary advice and monitoring she was performing in her private cardiology practice, could successfully treat patients with heart disease, weaning them off medications. This is extremely inexpensive for the patients, but is a threat to the income streams of cardiologists, hospitals, and pharmaceutical companies who treat the disease with medicines, operations, and recurring visits that create massive profits. Dr. Dulaney was surprised to find that fellow doctors responded "what would we do if we cured everyone of heart disease?"[38] A sick heart patient, continuing an unhealthy diet, can generate income for many years. Almost half of the U.S. population has cardiovascular disease, and the rate increases every year. Each year, over 950,000 people in the United States undergo an angioplasty to widen a narrowed coronary artery, usually with a stent, a wire mesh tube, left inside the artery to keep it open. This procedure costs about $30,000, adding up to a national annual total of $28 billion.[39] Cardiologists, without eliminating the underlying diet that drives their patient's disease, can be confident that the patient will be back again and again, covered by insurance, perhaps for another stint, or more intensive procedures. Bypass surgery, where healthy arteries harvested typically from a patient's legs are grafted onto the heart to bypass blocked ones, is the most common type of heart surgery. More than 300,000 procedures are performed each year in the United States at an average cost of over $120,000.[40] That's just about half the median price of a home! In total, bypass surgeries generate another $36 billion per year. If your heart condition deteriorates enough, you can get a new one. About 2,000 heart transplants are done in the U.S. a year and billable at a cost of about $1.4 million each, or $2.8 billion in total.[41] At well over $500 billion per year, treating cardiovascular disease is the number one healthcare expense in the United States. Expenses are projected to double in just the next 15 years to over $1 trillion.[42]

Today my brother Brett is an air ambulance helicopter pilot based in Colorado, covering a territory of the wide-open plains of Colorado and Nebraska, at the heart of American beef production. After many years in the Air Force flying search-and-rescue missions in the Rocky Mountains, shuttling commanders and politicians around Washington D.C., and a year in war training the Afghanistan Air Force to fly giant Russian choppers, the serenity of the plains has been a welcome respite. However, the action he sees is still intense. When called, he and a team of paramedics and nurses will buzz into the air and speed out into the plains to pick up patients living far away from hospitals. With hundreds of rescue flights in the past couple years, he has witnessed many people on the absolute worst day of their lives. Car accidents, falls, burns, severed limbs, and drug overdoses. Families killed. Mothers lost. However, of all the flights they are called on, the most common are for cardiovascular disease. Heart attacks or strokes account for about 40% of all his patients flown. With a cost of $25,000 to $80,000 per flight, cardiovascular disease is the bread and butter of helicopter rescues, and I'll bet it is the same for ambulances rolling and wailing throughout streets across our nation.

There are many highly profitable medications to act as a band-aid on the underlying dietary cause of heart disease. The number-one prescribed medication in the U.S. is Atorvastatin, commonly known by the brand name Lipitor.[43] It is used to treat high cholesterol and triglyceride levels, which may reduce the risk of angina, stroke, heart attack, and other heart and blood vessel problems. Over its lifetime of sales, Lipitor generated over $140 billion for the drug giant Pfizer, and still generates billions annually after its patent expired and competition exploded from generics. The third leading pharmaceutical is Lisinopril, also known as Prinivil or Zestril, which is used to treat high blood pressure and heart failure, reducing the risk of death after a heart attack. Millions of Americans take blood thinners, generating tens of billions in sales.[44] My mom was one of them. It was central to the reason she died bleeding out of her nose and mouth, alone in bed.

A lot of money is made producing and treating the consequences of our animal and processed-food diets. It is at the heart of so many of our anguished deaths. It is also at the very core of why we are losing some of the most amazing forms of life on our planet.

Chapter 5: **Our Earthcare Crisis**

When I first heard the rattlesnake buzzing, my body felt it was very close. The heartbeat in my ears was the only other sound my mind could process. The rasping rattle was hard for my eyes or ears to pinpoint, but I could see from the focused look of my gray-haired professor standing a few steps away that it was in his sight, hidden within striking distance from me in thick brush.

"Don't move. He's right there," he whispered.

I had been scanning all around me, but I had missed it repeatedly. A large eastern diamondback was curled up just in front of me, but it took the eyes of an expert, someone who has watched wildlife closely for years to see the patterns of nature. When my mind formed the image of the snake for the first time, less than 2 feet away, all the hair on my body stood on end – even though I was wearing snakebite-proof boots and shields to my knees. I slowly stepped back.

"Beautiful," Doc whispered as he gently, slowly coaxed it with a very long set of tongs and placed it softly into a portable cage.

Later placing my hands on that same angry-looking serpent for the first time made my nerves fire fast, my mind focused, even though its head was slipped into a protective tube to prevent bites and its body temperature purposefully lowered with ice to sedate it. Its smooth scaled skin was cool to the touch.

Its bold color pattern was striking against a black laboratory benchtop, but was stunning in its ability to camouflage itself in nature. Performing minor surgery on the animal to install a radio-tracking device and then later releasing it was the experience that taught me early on how cool the "study of life" could be, fostered in me by Dr. George Dalrymple, a very demanding, cantankerous, and often profanely yelling professor. He also enjoyed sipping whiskey and catching alligators, and being his assistant was nerve-racking but always filled with adventures. He opened my mind to ecology – learning how organisms interact with one another and the environment around them – and I finished an undergraduate program and master's degree learning about the web of life in the Everglades.

I slipped into its depths day and night catching salamanders, fish, alligators, and snakes – exploring places no one has probably ever been and witnessing serene, glorious moments waist deep in the slowly moving liquid life at the heart of Florida. I waded into alligator holes, was bitten thousands of times by mosquitoes, attacked by an entire nest of paper wasps, and struck in my snake-proof chaps by poisonous cottonmouths. I was once painfully blinded by a phasmid, a walking-stick insect, that sprayed a mace-like chemical into my eyes when I lifted it for a closer view. When its blast of mist seared me with burning pain, my first instinct, after a minute of shock and terror, was to rinse my eyes out. Unfortunately, on that day of fieldwork I had for the first time filled my water bottle with lemonade. It took nearly 10 minutes of crying, dripping snot, drooling, and spitting to get the chemical out and my wits back. The insect was nowhere to be seen, having escaped during his chemical defense and my fumbling to regain my senses. The River of Grass amazed me with its serene, yet often harsh, beauty. Life flourished in a very tough environment.

However, my own favorite experience in nature came a few years later when I was employed as a young marine biologist. While starting a Ph.D. during my mid-20s, I was hired as a research assistant to manage a conditions and trends study of the seagrass beds of the newly established Florida Keys National

Marine Sanctuary. My partner, Braxton, and I were given scuba gear, a credit card for fuel, and keys to a Jeep, behind which we could tow several types of boats from Florida International University. Our job was to launch at points from Key Largo to Key West, spend a day running out to a list of random GPS points, diving to the bottom and recording the types and amount of seagrass and algae that we found along transects we laid out. We were the first pioneers to visually map what was there. I felt like an astronaut exploring an unknown liquid world of blue and green that undulated like wind-blown prairies under cloudless skies. We also established permanent sampling locations we visited every three months so that seagrass growth and health could be monitored over time. Occasionally a large boat with a galley, bunks, and a captain would take us out for a week's worth of continuous diving, including long journeys with dive points scattered all the way out to the Dry Tortugas, 70 miles west of Key West.

Braxton and I did many hundreds of dives together, and we could communicate and joke effortlessly like brothers underwater. When the job became tedious, we enjoyed sneaking up on one another to clamp our hands, fingers jutting out like teeth of a predator, onto the others' unsuspecting leg. The scream and flurry of bubbles was hilariously terrifying during long days of serious data collection. Many days were incredibly fulfilling, but winter diving was often miserable. Temperatures in the shallow waters of the backcountry of the lower Keys could drop into the mid to low 50s. On many days of jumping into and out of that shocking water and frigid cold-front air, the most enjoyable moments became those when you peed in your wetsuit, the warmth slowly and gently creeping up your spine to hug you for a few far too brief minutes.

Every dive brought a new discovery of life. Tiny seahorses hidden among the grass blades. Dolphins encircling us with their trills of clicks. An octopus climbing up my arm to hide under my buoyancy device. Staring eye to eye with a wise cuttlefish, an electric kaleidoscope of colors constantly changing and dancing in waves across its skin, sending an alien message that I could not decipher. Green sea turtles munching paths through seagrass like lawnmowers. However, the animals I always wanted to see most were almost never seen: sharks. Well, except for nurse sharks, brown slumbering beasts living on the bottom and common as dogs. Often, when our day of work diving ended, we would speed off to the nearest coral reef and use a last tank of air to take in the radiance of the ecosystem and all its inhabitants. The colors and action of a reef are dazzling and constant. We dove every named reef in the Florida Keys, and endless small patch reefs for which none existed. In all those dives over several years, I never saw a shark other than a nurse shark. Not once.

Shark populations have been declining for a hundred years in the Keys, overfished along with many other finned species. In the early to mid-1900s, a factory in the Florida Keys reported processing 100 sharks per day, mainly to extract vitamin A.[45] Today, it can take days of fishing with 10-20 sampling lines deployed for scientists to encounter a single large shark. Two of the most common open ocean species of the region, silky sharks and oceanic whitetips, have declined by 90% and 99%, respectively.[46] Sharks have been decimated all over the world.[47] They have been living on our planet for 400 million years. They have survived five mass extinction events. They outlived dinosaurs. And they are key to maintaining healthy reefs and oceans. Top-down predation is well understood by ecologists to be a force that keeps many ecosystems in balance, reefs included. The reefs of the Florida Keys are a shadow of what they were only 50 years ago. They are struggling, unhealthy, and increasingly covered in algae. Corals, like elkhorn and staghorn, used to grow in stands that covered acres. Today only scattered remnants remain. Missing sharks are just one piece of the Jenga stack that has been removed. The ecosystems that remain are depleted and teetering.

At the end of a day's work running out transects in seagrass, Braxton and I decided to do something different. It was a calm and sunny summer afternoon, with no wind blowing or waves rolling. We had finished our dives early and still had extra air. We throttled the boat and headed southeast, watching the reefs pass behind us, the color of the water blending through dozens of shades of blue, from bright aquamarine to a deep endless azure. Land soon shrank into a small dark sliver on the horizon. We reached water that was over 500 feet deep, well into the Gulf Stream. It is a giant flowing river of warm water that swirls up from the Caribbean, hugs the coast of Florida, the U.S. east coast, and then turns east, eventually bathing England with a warmth that makes its high latitude climate much more enjoyable. After cutting the engine and gliding to a stop, we dropped the anchor over the side, lowering it to about 80 feet. It dangled, tiny, and far above the depths. The ocean was flat and clear as glass. Jumping in for a first "blue water" dive is heart pounding, especially for anyone like myself with an innate fear of heights. After the first splash, you look down, your arms and legs knowing there is nothing of substance below or around you to grab onto, nothing but primal salty liquid. Swimming feels so surreal, uncertain, poised above that blue, yet elevated by the fluid force from which my own being arose, stirred into action eons ago. This was Ocean. The origin of life.

After slowly descending down to the anchor, we both let go of the line, separated, and kicked away into the great blue. Only astronauts who have done space walks truly know what it feels like to be untethered from the limiting interaction of gravity and solid surfaces, but a deep blue dive is probably about as close as you can come on Earth. It quickly becomes disorienting. With no solid reference point other than the motionless anchor and the tiny hull far above, your mind's ability to determine size becomes unreliable. In normal surroundings, we gauge objects relative to others around. When nothing but clear blue water is around, my mind interpreted the first silvery fish I saw as being a foot in length, but when they swam close past my hand, they had shrunk to inches. I laughed bubbles in amazement. As Einstein so eloquently theorized, all things are relative. When I later glimpsed a large dark figure approaching out of magnificent blue, my mind rationally told me the object was probably smaller than my mind was tricking me into thinking. Then I saw it swim a large, slow curve beyond Braxton. It was much bigger than him, with far more girth. We both instinctively headed for the only semblance of safety, that 3-foot-long anchor dangling on a half-inch-thick rope. Braxton's eyes were wide and white, and his bubbles poured out in quicker bursts. I heard my own air rasping and bubbling faster. Slowly circling around us was a massive shark.

We knew our sharks. This was a bull shark, ranked among the top three most deadly by recorded fatal attacks along with great white sharks and tiger sharks. It circled slowly, its back arched. It stayed within 20 yards, and for a few heart-pounding minutes, its black eyes stared at us and we back at it. To be potential prey is humbling. Exhilarating. Then, as calmly as it had arrived, it disappeared into the blue. It was one of the most amazing moments of my life. Just as I had lacked context for comparing the size of organisms encountered in the great open blue ocean, most people have limited experience or knowledge about biodiversity and ecosystems as a background against which to see the true effects our diets and lifestyles are having on life that supports us. Examining the trends – the historical numbers of animals that once existed, their current status, and future prospects – will hopefully give an appreciation for what could quickly slip through our hands into extinction.

Life on Earth is astounding. As far as we know, our blue planet is the only place to harbor it, nurture it, evolve it. At the top of our planet's food chains are the big powerful predators that have always filled us with fear and awe. Lions, tigers, cougars, bears, wolves, sharks, and whales. They command our respect, but not enough of our consideration, and certainly not enough protection. Most people are unaware of the critical state of most of the world's predators. The 31 largest terrestrial carnivores include big cats, wild dogs, sea otters, bears, and hyenas. Of these, over half are listed by the International Union for the Conservation of Nature (IUCN) as threatened (vulnerable, endangered, or critically endangered) and are at risk of local or total extinction. Over three-quarters are undergoing continuing population declines, and they currently occupy on average less than half of the historical areas they occupied.[48] Marine predators are experiencing massive declines as well. Recent estimates suggest that populations of the largest sharks off Australia, including hammerhead, whaler, tiger, and white sharks have declined by 74-92% since the 1960s.[49] Stocks of blue and white marlin in the Atlantic, graceful top fish predators, are at 25% of historic levels, and their typical size has decreased from giants weighing many hundreds of pounds to around 50 pounds.[50] Global whale populations have been truly decimated. The largest animal to have ever lived in the billions of years of life on our planet, the Antarctic subspecies of blue whale, survives with only about 1% of its pre-whaling numbers remaining.[51] In terms of population decline, that would be the equivalent of killing every single person in the United States except those living in San Diego County.

A step down in terrestrial and aquatic food chains exhibits a similarly astounding loss of life. Of the 74 largest terrestrial herbivore species on Earth, about 60% are threatened with extinction. Twenty-five of these species examined in detail occupy only 19% of their historical ranges, and many – like elephant, hippopotamus, and black rhinoceros – occupy just tiny fractions of their historical areas.[52] In the ocean, the average state of global fish stocks is poor and declining. Nearly one in four marine fisheries collapsed during the period 1950–2000.[53] Numbers of fish and the size of fish are growing smaller and smaller.[54] The rate of decline of vertebrate populations is even higher in freshwaters than in terrestrial or marine realms. Freshwater megafauna, animals that can reach a body mass $\geq$30 kg (66 lbs) have experienced population declines of 88% from 1970 to 2012, with numbers of mega-fish declining by 95%.[55] In 2020, the giant Yangtze paddlefish, a species that lived on this planet alongside the dinosaurs, was finally declared extinct.[56] It hasn't been seen since 2003. It grew to 23 feet and 1,000 pounds, roughly the size of five human adults combined! A majestic ancient beast now gone forever. Like so many of the mega-species that are disappearing, we were just scratching the surface of understanding and appreciating the roles of these giants in our ecosystems and the benefits they provided us.

We are losing not just the megafauna from our lands, waterways, and oceans, but endless species that you have never heard of, and uncounted numbers that have never even been discovered before being erased from our planet. Bizarrely unique orchids, ferns, trees, frogs, birds, fishes, insects, worms, and on and on. We are in the midst of a great extinction event, on par with the asteroid strike that wiped out the dinosaurs. Organismal diversity encompasses the full taxonomic hierarchy of life and its components, from individuals upwards to populations, subspecies and species, genera, families, phyla, and beyond to kingdoms and domains. The amount of organismal diversity is astounding. A handful of healthy soil may contain 8 million prokaryotic species, microscopic organisms without a nucleus like bacteria.[57] Many millions of prokaryote species likely exist. Even smaller, trillions of types of viruses may exist.[58] Of the eukaryotes, the higher animals like plants, insects, and animals, only about 1.9 million are known and described.[59] Scientists have had lower and upper estimates of a few million to more than 100 million, and a recent working figure of around 8.7 million species[60] – about the same number of prokaryotes found in a handful of soil! Life is full of surprises. No one knows how many types of organisms we have, and we discover and describe them very slowly. New species are being described at a rate of about 18,000 per year.[61] At that rate, it will take over 300 years to describe the at least 6 million more we think might exist.

However, we are losing these species faster than they can even be discovered. It is estimated that we have encountered and described about 80% of the planet's mammals, birds, fishes, and plants, but only 30% of the crabs and other crustaceans, 20% of the insects and spiders, 6% of the fungi, and less than 1% of the prokaryotes.[62] In the Amazon, scientists think that there are at least 11,000 more tree species out there that have never been discovered that we know absolutely nothing about.[63] That is over 10 times more species of trees than found in all of North America. How fast are we losing species before we can discover them? It is impossible to know the extinction rate for most groups of species. If we don't even know how many species exist, how can we hope to know how many are going extinct? Various estimates range from a few thousand to more than 100,000 species being extinguished every year.[64] Scientists estimate the background natural extinction rate, calculated from fossils. Somewhere between one in 10 million to one in a million species should go extinct every year.[65] If we roughly estimate the number of eukaryote species on earth at 10 million, that means between one and 10 are estimated to naturally go extinct a year, which is about the same rate new species are theorized to be created through evolution.

One of the best studied groups of animals can give us a hint of how much the extinction rate has changed in the presence of humans.[66] Birds have long fascinated us, they are relatively easy to spot, and have been well examined by scientists and citizens alike. An estimated 10,000-12,000 species of birds exist today. At the background rate, it would be expected that a single bird species would go extinct somewhere between a high rate of one every 100 years and a low rate of one every 1,000 years. However, once humans arrived, birds rapidly declined in numbers. The Polynesian Islands provide a good place to examine what is happening. Up to an estimated 1,000 species of birds were driven extinct from Pacific islands by the arrival of the Polynesians.[67] Many were truly amazing. The moa were nine species of flightless bird endemic to New Zealand. The two largest species reached about 3.6 m (~12 ft) in height with neck outstretched, twice the height of modern ostriches, and weighed about 230 kg (>500 lbs). The moa disappeared from Earth by the 1800s, about 600 years after the first Polynesians arrived there. Human colonization of the Hawaiian Islands led to the extinction of more than 50% of native bird species.[68] Globally, the extinction rate for birds is estimated to be 100 times the natural rate, and is likely going to increase dramatically. Over 1,100 bird species, which is greater than 10% of all birds, are listed as critically endangered, endangered, or vulnerable.[69] If all these species go extinct in the next 100 years, that equates to 1,000 times the natural background rate. The factors that have placed more than 1,000 birds to date at risk of disappearing forever do not yet even include the coming effects of climate change. Many groups of organisms are far more threatened than birds. Over 20% of mammals, 30% of reef-building corals, 40% of amphibians, and 50% of freshwater mussels are threatened.[69] We are most likely wiping species off the face of the planet at least 1,000 times faster, with some scientists estimating 10,000 times faster, than nature does.[70]

However, it is not just the diversity of organisms, like birds, that we are losing at an increasing rate but also the diversity of the ecosystems within which they live. The unique assemblages of plants, animals, and their interaction with water, energy, and nutrients is what makes our planet livable. Rainforests hold and slowly release clean water for people to drink, the coral reefs produce fish that feed us, and mangrove forests protect shorelines and provide food and habitat for those fish – even species like massive barracuda – when they are only inch-long juveniles. Ecosystems support the incredible biodiversity of life and provide services that give us life. Unfortunately, we are razing ecosystems all over the planet. We cut them down, pave them over, drain them, fill them in, plow them under, and pollute them with our waste and toxins. Approximately 75% of coral reefs worldwide are already lost, under imminent risk of collapse, or in grave danger of irreparable damage.[71] Reefs in the wider Caribbean have lost approximately 80% of the coral that covered their surfaces in the 1970s.[72] A healthy coral reef has at least 25% of its surface covered with live coral. In the Florida Keys, coral coverage on many reefs is now reduced to an alarming 2%.[73] Around Miami, we have destroyed 98% of the native pine forests outside of Everglades National Park.[74] In portions of Biscayne Bay, the shallow subtropical bay that lines the city's waterfront, over 75% of the seagrass has died off in just the last decade.[75] Many other ecosystems around the planet are just as highly threatened, if not more.

This massive loss of organisms and ecosystems – and the benefits they provide us through food, water, climate, and spiritual inspiration – represents only the fraction of biodiversity loss that we can see occurring before our very eyes. When I first snorkeled Biscayne Bay in 1990, it was a prairie of seagrass waving under vibrant and clear water through which I could see about 100 feet. The aquamarine waters provided the picture-perfect background for the downtown skyline and the TV show *Miami Vice*. Photosynthesis churned so powerfully in the summer that oxygen rose in bubbly streams from its blades. It was like swimming through crystal clear champagne. It was full of schools of bonefish, spotted eagle rays, horseshoe crabs, and lobster. Today those same places are now a murky, brown mess filled with algae into which I can often barely see a few feet, and in which I rarely find any animals swimming or crawling. However, as we lose ecosystems and the species within them, we also lose something that our eyes cannot fathom – the biodiversity found within the species. We are losing our planet's genetic diversity, the massive variety of coded information that makes life's operating system function. The more species we have, and the more individuals of a species, the more genetic diversity we have. Discovering and understanding the operating system of different species has brought us some of the most incredible advances in human ingenuity. We are just beginning to scratch the surface of what this information could do to make human life better. A shining example of a life form and its unique genetic makeup that dramatically helped and advanced mankind comes from one of the lowest life forms, a species among the single-celled prokaryotes.[76]

Discovered in 1969 in a scalding spring in Yellowstone National Park, *Thermus aquaticus*, is a species of bacteria that can tolerate temperatures so high that they would normally cook an organism's proteins. You can see the effect of high temperature on proteins when an egg white solidifies as you cook it. Proteins run most processes in cells, and high temperatures are usually fatal. However, *Thermus aquaticus* evolved to survive within scalding heat, which made it incredibly useful. Taq polymerase, a heat-tolerant protein derived from this organism, is at the root of the entire field of modern genetics, forensics, cancer treatments, and crop breeding. These technologies, and many more, are dependent on making many copies of DNA from a small amount of starter DNA. We can take DNA from one single cell and make millions and millions of copies, giving scientists enough material to study patterns. This replication of DNA occurs via the polymerase chain reaction (PCR), which is a reaction that is performed millions of times a day in labs all over the world to examine crime scenes, grow rice that prevents blindness, and determine who your relatives might be. PCR requires the DNA sample to be heated up to high temperatures, which prior to the discovery of Taq polymerase, destroyed all the proteins that are needed to copy the DNA. Discovering *Thermus aquaticus*, and uncovering its own unique genetic code that produced a protein, Taq polymerase, which could replicate DNA under high temperatures, unlocked a genetics-driven future for human society that is still in its infancy. That lowly prokaryote will dramatically alter our future. With only less than 1% of all prokaryote species discovered, we are destined to discover equally revolutionary services from its species diversity and underlying genetic diversity.[77] That is, if we don't destroy them first.

The global human population increases by 85 million people each year, which is equivalent to doubling the entire U.S. population in under four years. We are expected to reach 9 billion people by 2050 and stabilize somewhere between 9 and 11 billion individuals.[78] We are an incredible species unique in our intelligence and technological capacity. We have stood on the moon. We have split the atom. We can see back in time. We can predict the future. We have created artificial intelligence. But we are undermining the very natural systems that make our life on this planet beautiful, bountiful, and possible. Through the loss of majestic predators, the erasing of millions of acres of biodiverse tropical forests, and the destruction of vibrant coral reefs around the globe, we are snuffing out, on a gargantuan scale, the very thing that created us: life. The amazing diversity of life is what led to our evolution and existence, and it has provided us with food, water, shelter, and a sense of awe since the very beginning. The advancements and choices we have been making during the past few hundred years have given us tremendous benefits, but threaten to undermine us. I am an optimist. I believe we have the intelligence to recognize our faults, to learn better options, and to steer our planet and ourselves into a bountiful future where people and nature are more in harmony, benefiting from each other – a mutualism.

Although our enormous and growing population size is the ultimate cause of our planetary change, one activity we all do multiple times a day is the primary driver of our biodiversity loss, soil loss, water pollution, climate change, and overall ecological degradation. The primary driver of our earthcare crisis is also the main cause of our healthcare crisis. It's the food we choose to put in our mouths.

Chapter 6: **Pura Vida**

Costa Rica. What do you imagine when you hear the name? Cascading waterfalls, misty cloud forests, smoldering volcanoes, and towering vine-draped trees? Monkeys, toucans, sloths, and jaguars? The images of Costa Rica we see are of stunning beauty. They beckon you to come for a visit, to unwind, and get lost among the rhythms of a pure life. The country is a prime example of a country that has protected its natural wonders, a bastion of peaceful democracy, and a sustainable-energy example for the rest of the world to follow. It may very well be on your bucket list of places to visit. It's the kind of place we dream of going for the ultimate escape into tropical beauty. The last thing that comes to your mind when you picture that emerald and cyan colored nation is cows. Cows? Yes, cows. They rule over Costa Rica, as they do throughout much of our planet.

My first trip to Costa Rica was in the summer of 1990, a year after exploring the Colombian Amazon. That itch to see more of the world had become a raging fever. I wanted to immerse myself again in a foreign world, to live among a different language and see the extravagance of nature in more forms. After losing my college scholarship during my freshman year, I was forced to return to live again with my parents and attend college back in Ohio. That winter was absolutely miserable. Cold, gray, and depressing. I just wanted to escape back to warmth and sunshine. The Cleveland Zoo became my respite, especially the steamy rainforest exhibit, which I would regularly choose to spend a few hours exploring, instead of attending lectures. However, as fate would determine, I did attend my Spanish class the day a guest speaker from Amigos de las Americas appeared and told us stories of adventure awaiting. Amigos is like a mini Peace Corps, where as a volunteer you spend two months over summer, instead of two years, in a developing foreign country helping support community health and education efforts. I was immediately drawn to the journey in a strange land among another culture. I liked the idea of helping people I believed were less fortunate than I. That summer, after several months of training and fundraising, I was off to Costa Rica. When I arrived, I learned I would be assigned to work in a small town on the Pacific Coast. I would live with a local family, immersed in their lives, assigned to work on a school restoration project.

The journey from the capital, San Jose, to my destination took two days. First, a bus ride out of the cooler mountains on a windy paved two-lane highway to an evening's rest in a hot and humid town with horses and cowboys on the plains of the Pacific. The next day's travels started with a three-hour metal-and-bone-rattling ride on a much older bus across dirt and gravel roads that alternated between a moonscape of potholes and a washboard of erosion. The bus was stiflingly humid and packed with people, goods, and clucking chickens. This was a bus ride I would take many times to and from my town, and it was an adventure in itself. On one trip, a woman laid a piece of newspaper down in the aisle and plopped her toddler son onto it, stripped naked except for his little faded yellow t-shirt. He smiled, squatted down, and pooped on the paper. With a nonchalant crinkling, she balled up the deposit, and tossed it out the window. No one but me even noticed. However, during that first journey out toward the coast, my eyes were largely fixed on the world passing by the vibrating, rain-streaked, steamy window. What I remember most were fences, lush green fields, cowboys, and the cattle they herded. The same angular white Brahman cattle that

I saw in the Amazon. On several occasions, the bus had to pause its journey, waiting for a herd to finish passing across the road before us, a couple of cowboys coaxing them on. Sometimes, the bus would come to a full stop, honking its horn, trying to budge cows blocking the road, untended and uninterested in moving in the tropical heat.

As the bus journeyed on, its seats gradually emptied as people got off under big shady trees next to rustic wood and tin roof houses that occasionally appeared along the route. I would get off at the last stop, along with my partner for the summer, and the supervisor from Amigos that would help get us settled with our family. However, our stop was still more than a two-hour walk from our final destination, as it was at the edge of a bridgeless river too wide and deep for the bus to pass. The three of us stripped off our boots and carried them and our backpacks across the muddy river. We did that two more times before reaching the town. In 1990, Ostional was isolated and undeveloped, a tiny cluster of houses tucked just behind a mile-long black beach pounded by the relentless surf of the grand Pacific Ocean. During the entire two months I was there, only a handful of trucks passed through, those big enough to cross the natural moats that kept most motorists away. Travel was primarily by foot or horse. The family I lived with was the only one with electricity, which only came on during the early evening for an hour or two, powering a handful of lights and a TV for watching soccer, all brought to life from an old chugging diesel generator in the yard. We were also one of the only houses with running water, which flowed as long as there was enough water in the uphill stream from which it was shunted. I had to filter it with a purifier before I drank it. Even so, I eventually was struck with an intestinal illness, enough to keep me shitting and throwing up for several miserable, groaning days. It was likely contaminated with livestock waste upstream.

Normally, each morning just after sunrise, I spent time working at the school. With Amigos' help and nearby carpenters, restrooms with flush toilets were being installed. Someone had to dig the giant hole by hand into which the septic holding tank would be constructed. That someone was my Amigos partner and me. In the tropics, manual labor can only be done during a few morning hours, before the heat becomes unbearable, making it unhealthy to do much of anything except rest in the shade. Those morning hours were already brutally hot and humid. It took many weeks to dig that hole. The afternoons were spent studying Spanish, exploring the beach, and sometimes hunting in the shady forests with my Costa Rican brothers.

We hunted mainly to augment the staple meal we ate three times a day, beans and rice. Every single day for those two months, breakfast, lunch, and dinner was a plate of beans and rice, sometimes placed side by side, or with the beans in their sauce plopped on top of the rice, or mixed together and served as *gallo pinto*, translated as "spotted chicken." A meal sometimes included an egg. Or salad, which consisted of finely sliced raw cabbage with a squeeze of lime juice. Occasionally it would come with a small piece of chicken on the bone, from the many birds that scratched around the yard, and a drizzle of spiced sauce made from their fatty rendering. On rare occasions, we had a small piece of beef. Like barbecue sauce as a kid, I learned to douse the increasingly boring beans and rice in Lizano, the brown tangy bottled sauce found on every dining table in Costa Rica. After the first two weeks, I stopped caring about how it all tasted. I began to look at a meal not for pleasure, but just for sustenance and energy. Fuel in the tank. Physical labor in the hot tropics emptied the tank fast. This is how the majority of people on our planet look at food. My body grew lean and ripped.

Hunting for bush meat became a primal pleasure. We donned masks and scouted nearby river bottoms for crayfish. We knocked large lizards out of nearby trees with rocks, provoking the family dog, Osito, to make the final thrashing kill. "Little Bear," that foot-tall black-and-white friend, was also adept at tracking down and chasing armadillos in the forest, cornering them in their burrows. Twenty minutes of digging with a machete, and a final stab, rendered the soon-to-be meal lifeless. Those delicious treats of meat, cooked over a wood fire, were revered by all. But the most unique treat, one which most people have never consumed, sustained me regularly throughout much of that summer: sea turtle eggs. I ate them fried, hard boiled, scrambled, as omelets, and raw. They are a poor, thick, and slightly fishy replacement for chicken eggs. But during the summer, they were available in astronomical numbers on the beach just steps from my door.

Ostional is one of the last places on Earth that still hosts a true spectacle of nature, one on par with the great millions-strong wildebeest migrations of the Serengeti. Olive ridley sea turtles gather from across the Pacific to lay eggs on Ostional Beach. Weeks before nesting, a "flotilla" of increasing numbers of turtles congregates close offshore. I was warned against swimming in the ocean, which I did only a handful of times, not because of the continuous massive pounding surf, but because large tiger sharks were always patrolling for a turtle meal. Prompted by some innate signal, the *arribada*, or arrival, begins. At first, a few hundred turtles will come out on the beach, followed by a steady stream of thousands of animals for the next several days and up to a week. During an arribada in the rainy season, when I was there, hundreds of thousands of turtles crawl ashore, dig nests, and deposit up to 10 million eggs.[79]

I witnessed two arribadas, and they were otherworldly. Turtles fill nearly every available space on the beach, crawling, digging, plopping out golf-ball-sized eggs. The air is thick with wet reptilian odor. The arribadas started late in the day with a high tide and continued all night long. I never slept while it happened. I ended up alone, the only human soul walking among tens of thousands of animals whose ancestors have been doing this for hundreds of millions of years. A moment like that under a Milky Way arcing across the black sky puts one's tiny life and concerns in perspective among the eons of time and millions of strange and beautiful beasts that have called this little blue planet home. When I returned to town at sunrise, I passed a couple of the armed guards that protected the beach from poachers who would try to sneak in and steal eggs. They smiled. Everyone in town knew who the Amigos from the Americas were.

Just as I thought I would return to my bed for some much-needed rest, the entire town was gathering and heading out to the beach. I followed, and soon I was elbow deep in the sand helping gather eggs. Ostional is the only beach in the world where harvesting turtle eggs is legal. Ecologists studying the olive ridleys discovered that most of the eggs deposited in the first few nights of an arribada are destroyed by other turtles coming later to dig their nests. Millions of broken shells are scattered across the black sands. Black vultures and crabs feast on them. Therefore, the government of Costa Rica allows the community of Ostional to harvest the eggs on the first three days of an arribada. In return, the villagers protect the turtles with watchful patrols day and night. Most of the eggs are sold and distributed around the country, where they are consumed raw in bars along with a shot of liquor, believed to increase male vitality. It is near certain that consuming a turtle egg will not aid a desired or sustained hard-on in any way. However, I am certain that seeing tens of thousands of nesting adults, followed about 45 days later by millions of baby sea turtles erupting from their nests, will lift anyone's spirits with excitement and passion for life.

Costa Rica during that first visit seemed to me like a safe harbor for nature, a country that valued wildlife as its primary resource. I love the country and its people deeply, and always will. For the next 10 years, I returned every summer to visit my family in Ostional. I had discovered that they were, in many important ways, much more fortunate than I. During that decade, I hitchhiked and rode lots of jarring buses to explore all corners of the nation's natural beauty. However, the more I learned about the earthcare crisis facing our planet, the more I saw the details of how Costa Rica had been equally decimated. During the 1980s, the decade just before I arrived, Costa Rica had one of the world's highest deforestation rates, and only about one-quarter of its forests remained.[80] Its beauty was so stunning and the journey so exhilarating, that during those early years, I never realized what a role those cowboys and cattle played in the country's transformation. If any animal best represented Costa Rica, it was not the sloth, jaguar, or monkey. It was the cow.

One might think even a banana could be a better symbol. After tourism, bananas have been a top income-generating industry. The first export plantations, among the first in the world, were established there in the late 1800s.[81] The country is ranked among the leaders in the world for banana exports.[82] Anyone who has traveled to the east side of Costa Rica has driven highways with enormous stretches where rainforest was converted to miles and miles of repetitive rows of cloned banana plants. However, when it comes to land use, people cleared forests for cows far more than bananas, or anything else. By the time I first visited Costa Rica, pasture used for livestock covered just under half of the entire country's land. Thankfully, that number has dropped to around one-quarter of the country as many pastures have been reforested. Today about half the country is covered in forests, split roughly between untouched primary forest and secondary regrowth or plantation forests. National parks cover 10% of the country, but with other types of protected areas such as forestry reserves and wetlands, about one-quarter of the country is under some form of land protection. Cattle, totaling approximately 1.5 million head, now occupy more than twice as much land as national parks and as much land as all protected natural areas combined. Amazingly, the combined weight of all the country's cattle is four times more than that of all the Costa Ricans living there. It is still a country that prioritizes cows.

However, cattle not only use tremendous amounts of land in this incredibly biodiverse country, a nation comparable to South Carolina or Kentucky in territory and population size, but they produce very little food for people. Compared to bananas, the numbers are striking. Bananas are grown on only 1% of Costa Rica's land, producing about 2.6 billion kg of the yellow fruits. About 78 million kg of beef and 1.1 billion kg of milk are produced from the cows feeding on one-quarter of all the country's land.[82] This equates to twice as much food being produced from bananas using 25 times less land. As beef and milk cost more and can generate more income per kilogram, one might think they offer a better financial return. However, this potential logic also fails for cattle. Bananas generate 25% more value (>$1 billion vs. $760 million) from 25 times less land than the products generated from cattle. Admittedly, bananas are not a good example of sustainable agriculture. They are heavily sprayed with pesticides and feed mainly foreign countries. One may argue that the cattle pasture that generated beef and milk is far more important than land growing bananas because cattle produce protein that people need, and bananas produce none. It is true that bananas produce no protein, but there are plants that do, and in much higher concentrations and far more efficiently than cattle.

One of the most amazing and nutritious crops that people have eaten for thousands of years are soybeans. Not just enjoyed as tofu, tempeh, or soymilk, which is integral to many east Asian cultures, but cooked fresh, dried and roasted, sprouted, or ground into flour and integrated into endless recipes and potential products. It is a powerhouse of nutrition and health benefits, a plant, like many legumes, that makes concentrated protein. Through the process of nitrogen fixation, accomplished through a symbiotic partnership with bacteria living on the plant's roots, soybeans can extract nitrogen gas directly from the atmosphere and convert it into protein concentrated in its beans. Pound for pound, soybeans contain 2.5 times more protein than lean ground beef and 10 times more protein than milk[83] – but without any of the saturated fats or cholesterol, the fuel for cardiovascular disease. Soybean protein is a complete plant protein, meaning it contains all of the amino acids essential for human health.[84] However, it is slightly lower in the key amino acids methionine and cystine, but these can be easily supplemented by eating brown rice, whole wheat, rye, or any other whole grains, which don't necessarily need to be eaten during the same meal as soy.

Studies have shown the health benefits of soy consumption, including decreasing LDL-cholesterol, improving insulin sensitivity, and reducing weight gain.[85] Men have jokingly replied to me that soy is high in estrogen and they have heard this might affect their testosterone levels, and even make their breasts grow. Soy contains phytoestrogens, which can improve health due to their protective effects on cardiovascular disease, positive effects on weight loss, reduction of breast and prostrate cancers, and strengthening of bones.[86] Soy can protect against several aspects of obesity and associated metabolic syndrome.[87] A meta-analysis of 32 studies published in 2010 reported that the consumption of isoflavones, a group of phytoestrogens common in soy, had no significant effect on circulating testosterone or free testosterone levels in men.[88] Many other studies have since produced similar results showing no negative effect of soy on male hormones, even as related to muscles and weight lifting.[89] However, obese men have lower testosterone levels.[90] A man is much more likely to grow larger drooping breasts, composed of fat, from eating a high-fat animal-product-centered diet, which drives obesity, than from consuming soy. Eating soy will drive the opposite effect.[91]

Land can produce far more soybeans than beef. On average, a hectare of pasture in Costa Rica is producing about 65 kg of beef and 1,000 kg of milk.[82] If it were instead producing soybeans, over 2,000 kg of the protein-packed legumes could be produced on the same hectare. Many farms in the world exceed 3,000 kg per hectare.[92] Due to the higher concentration in soybeans, if you compare the amount of protein produced, land converted from pasture to soybean could produce about 17 times more protein than current beef and milk production. If Costa Rica wanted to continue setting an example for the world with its impressive reforestation trend, it would shift its cattle industry to a soybean industry. If it converted completely and only produced 2000 kg per hectare, it would need to shift only about 6% of its pasture to soy production to produce about the same amount of protein as it does now from beef and milk, and could reforest the remaining 94% of its pastures.

Due to the innate production-magnifying power of plant-based protein, Costa Rica would require only 70,000 hectares, or about 1.5% of all its land to produce the same amount of protein as it currently milks and slaughters from cattle on 1.2 million hectares, one-quarter of all its land. Nearly three-quarters of Costa Rica could be covered in forest, as it was a hundred years ago. The ecotourism industry, which is the top money-maker for the country, would benefit from having more of the natural beauty that draws tourists. Increased water storage by more forests would benefit the hydropower industry, which generates over 75% of the nation's energy needs.[93] This is especially important given recent droughts affecting Costa Rica, which are projected to increase in the future.[94] Decreased erosion would improve conditions for downstream coral reefs. However, as this book will reveal, totally eliminating meat is not my recommendation or goal. We should leave a small portion for the cattle, to allow for an occasional beef treat during their revered barbecue celebrations, with the culture of Costa Rican cowboys and Lizano included.

Why can land produce so much more food or protein from growing crops than raising livestock? It's all about efficiency and energy loss. A basic tenet in ecology is that with every step you make up a food chain, you will lose about 90% of the energy from the previous lower step and retain only 10% in animal mass.[95] For example, if you had an area of land from which 10 people were supported by eating only plant-based food production, that same land could support only one person, at best, eating just cattle meat if you fed the cows all those same plants. This is because about 90% of the energy available in the plants is burned up by a cow being a cow, fueling its own metabolism, leaving only 10% to be converted into cow flesh and bones that is then consumed by a person. Roughly, land can support 10 times as many people who are vegan than strictly carnivore. The efficiency of energy conversion varies among livestock, with pigs and chickens being more efficient at converting plants to flesh. Cattle are by far the worst.

People have also tried to increase efficiencies by creating concentrated animal feeding operations (CAFOs) where animals are raised in highly unnatural and unhealthy hyper-concentrated numbers, crammed into far too small cages, packed together in high densities. This maximizes profits during production but also enables livestock to be raised closer to urban areas, concentrated for easy processing and shorter shipping distances. Again, this maximizes profits. This is the growing trend across the planet. In CAFOs, livestock are fed crops, antibiotics, and hormones to make them grow faster and better convert plant energy into flesh. Again, driven by increasing profits. Antibiotics not only foster faster growth, but are necessary to control disease, which can run rampant in such packed conditions. If most people visited these facilities, and followed the path of one of these animals from birth to slaughter, they would probably never want to eat its meat again. The conditions in these facilities are atrocious for the animals, and the industry fights very hard to prevent the public from seeing them. For example, pig's tails need to be trimmed off under these conditions because other stressed pigs will chew them off.[96] For similar reasons, chicken beaks are cut off, preventing them from pecking and cannibalizing each other.[97] Imagine if you were packed for your entire life with hundreds of people into a small room, never going outside to see sunshine, standing in everyone's urine and feces, constantly bumping into other people. It would get ugly fast. Your health would certainly suffer. In the U.S., it is illegal in some areas to secretly film and expose these facilities, for fear that the exposure could affect profits. Those profits hold great power over elected officials and the laws they pass. The overuse of antibiotics in livestock is also fostering the evolution of antibiotic-resistant strains of pathogens, meaning it will become more challenging to treat infections in people. Almost 80% of the antibiotics in the U.S. are taken not by people but by livestock! Americans use more antibiotics per kilogram of meat and poultry produced than any other developed country.[98]

Costa Rica does stand out as a positive example and should be recognized and commended for its commitment to peaceful democracy, education, protecting natural resources, conserving biodiversity, and maximizing renewable energy use. It is an emerald gem among nations, even with one-quarter of its land still dedicated to cattle. The reforestation trend that has occurred in Costa Rica during the past few decades is largely an anomaly in surrounding Latin America and the rest of the world. However, its increasing consumption of meat, other animal products, and processed foods is part of the ongoing diet trend around the globe, along with the ensuing obesity and all the associated health ailments.

The production of animal-based foods for humans continues to transform our planet like nothing else. Livestock production uses about 75% of all agricultural land that we have developed on Earth. Producing our animal-based food products uses about 30% of the ice-free land surface of the entire planet, making it the largest use of land by mankind.[99] If you add up the weight of all the plants, animals, and humans on the surface of our planet – the total terrestrial biomass – our livestock comprises one-fifth of all of it. Livestock biomass is twice that of humans. Livestock consume one-third of all the cereal crops we produce. This impact on the planet and its ecosystems is incredible. Thirty years ago, when I flew over the Amazon for the first time, I saw huge swaths of unbroken rainforest. Over time, that ecosystem, the largest tropical forest on our planet, has been increasingly chewed up – by livestock. Over 80% of deforested land in the Amazon was likely converted to pasture, though a portion been abandoned with some secondary forest regrowth occuring.[100] Much of the remaining deforested portion is increasingly covered by feed crops, like soybeans and corn, which are fed to livestock in CAFOs around the world. We are turning huge tracts of our most biodiverse regions, filled with thousands of plants and animal species, countless undiscovered, to enormous biological deserts inhabited by a few species of grasses, cows, and neat rows of a couple of animal feed crops. All this to increasingly make us fatter and unhealthier.

Ironically, Costa Rica produces minimal amounts of soybeans, but instead imports them, not for human consumption, but to feed to livestock in its CAFOs that produce chicken, pork, and farmed fish. These CAFOs have fueled a rapid increase in the amount of animal products that Costa Ricans eat, which has been fueled by a massive expansion of the

U.S.-branded fast-food industry into the country. When I first visited there in 1990, only a handful of fast-food outlets existed. I'd bet I could have counted them all on my two hands. Today there are hundreds, including over 50 McDonald's and over 50 Pizza Huts.[101] Because of the financial strength and marketing prowess of these companies, and the highly addictive nature of the unhealthy food they sell, Costa Rica has become a fast-food nation. And its health is suffering.

The traditional diet of beans, rice, fruit, and veggies augmented with a little chicken, pork, or beef, which flourished only a few decades ago, has quickly morphed into the animal-product and junk-food dietary pattern of Americans. Along with it has come the American pattern of increasing obesity, diabetes, and cardiovascular disease. Obesity among Costa Rica's population has increased by almost four times since the 1970s, from about 6% then to 24% today.[102] Diabetes has doubled. Although these rates are not as bad as in the United States, it has been sad to personally witness the changes that my country's culture and businesses have inflicted on Ticos, as Costa Ricans are warmly called. "Pura vida," the common phrase shared among Ticos and visitors alike to reflect their vibrant, beautiful nation and pure, natural life, has evolved year by year to be better described as a "vida gorda" – a fat life.

However, if Costa Ricans can be leaders in natural resource protection via reforestation, they certainly can also be leaders through healthy diet-driven conservation and health.

Chapter 7: **Eating the Earth**

When you pick up a hamburger, what choice are you making? First, you are choosing something delicious. Just the thought of perfectly charbroiled ground beef, nestled in a bun and topped perhaps with ketchup, mustard, onions, lettuce, and tomato will make most people's mouths start to water. Eating a burger is an American tradition that is driven overwhelmingly by one thing: It tastes great. It's fun. It just feels good. Same for pizza. I absolutely love eating both. But I also know very well what it does to my body and the planet. I know that I am at risk, like most people, for cardiovascular disease, perhaps even a little more. My mother passed away from complications tied to it. My father has been on high blood pressure medication most of his life, has suffered two heart attacks, and has undergone angioplasties for both. During my Ph.D., I read stacks of scientific papers and books about the effects of different diets on human health, and there is no doubt that for almost anyone, eliminating or greatly reducing the intake of animal products and processed foods will make them healthier and help them live longer. This extended lifespan will be measured not just in additional years but with that time being more mobile, active, and fulfilled. And able to see your own genitals. A diet dominated by plant-based whole foods is the key. If you match this healthier diet with regular exercise, your odds of living – and living better – are even better. Period.

People often point out to me relatives or friends that have lived into their 80s, 90s, or beyond who ate meat regularly their entire lives. Yes, there are always exceptions. Few choices in life are completely black or white. Most are shades of gray. Some people who drink heavily, smoke cigarettes, or snort cocaine for many decades can also live long lives. They all don't develop liver dysfunction, lung cancer, or emphysema, or destroy their nasal passages from long-term abuse. But most people will experience adverse consequences, especially if they gorge on them like we do now with animal-based foods. The average person will suffer from such self-abuse, and their lives will likely be shortened and certainly sapped of vitality. However, some people truly would rather burn out than fade away. Climbing mountains, big-wave surfing, or whitewater kayaking are all risky activities with the danger of an early death highly increased. It is everyone's right to treat their bodies how they would like and to put their life on the line. It is, after all, their life. Not yours. Not mine. If you or someone you know enjoys consuming meat by the pound, cheese by the block, junk food by the box, or five sodas a day, regardless of the consequences to their health, that is their choice. And their right. Just like it is the right of an MMA fighter to jump in a ring and fight, risking bodily harm or long-term debilitation that often comes from intense contact sports. However, keep in mind that eating like that also raises healthcare costs for us as a society and drives up the amount we all pay in insurance premiums and taxes required to support government programs like Medicare, which makes up 15% of our federal budget. As expected, cardiovascular disease, followed closely by diabetes, is the largest expense within public health programs.[103] That choice to gorge on unhealthy food also has costly environmental consequences. We all pay for each other's food choices, and coaxing others to eat better helps us all. If fewer people ate such poor diets, we would all get to keep more money in our pockets to spend. Perhaps on a vacation to a richly reforested Costa Rica.

For me, improving my own health was by far the most important factor in a decision to alter my diet. Call me selfish. At 50 years of age, I have less than 12% body fat, well-defined muscles, and six-pack abs. I take no medications. Other than a rickety shoulder and gray hair that seems to spread like a smoldering fire, I am in similar physical shape as I was in my early 20s. I weigh about 15 pounds more than I did as a senior in high school, 30 if you count what I had to cut down to during wrestling season for matches. I have been heavier a few times, and I know that strange, unpleasant feeling of tightened jeans and love-handles sprouting around my waist. I don't like that feeling. My back usually hurts. It's a canary in a coal mine telling me that I am not treating my body well. I know exactly what caused those unhealthy periods and the only thing I had to change to shed the pounds: the type of food I put in my mouth. Eating a diet heavily dominated by whole plant-based foods naturally and easily makes me thinner, gives me more energy, and makes exercise and my entire day easier. I just feel better all around. I am certain it will do the exact same for anyone else who makes a similar choice.

Consuming animal products affects personal and environmental health through a variety of pathways and mechanisms. Depending on what you eat and where you live, your choice to put flesh, eggs, dairy products, or processed junk foods into your diet, and how often, can have many different radiating and cascading effects both within your own body, but just as importantly, on the world around you. The key pathways through which eating animal products drives ecosystem degradation and biodiversity loss are summarized in the following diagram:

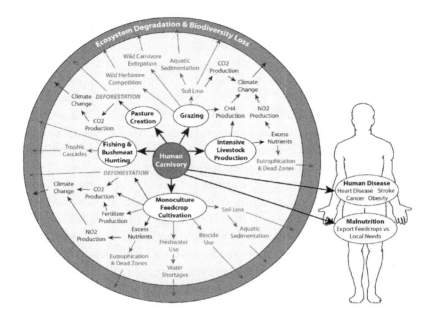

When you choose food that comes from animals, you affect our environment through one or more of five major pathways: (1) bushmeat hunting and fishing, (2) grazing, (3) pasture creation, (4) monoculture feed crop cultivation, or (5) intensive animal production. Several of these pathways are tied to and affect each other. Of course, human carnivory (eating animal products) drives human diseases like heart disease, strokes, obesity, and cancers. However, it can also contribute to malnutrition as developing countries will often prioritize export livestock or feed crop industries, using the productive soils and water they require at the expense of growing crops and supplying water for agriculture that feeds local, impoverished communities.[104]

~ Bushmeat Hunting and Fishing ~

When I was hunting crayfish, lizards, and armadillos or gathering turtle eggs in that first hungry summer in Costa Rica, it never dawned on me that I was participating in the oldest way of feeding oneself, a skill that goes back millions of years in our evolutionary history. I was hungry, it tasted great, and was incredibly rewarding. Deep within our psyche is an innate hunter's drive to find food and survive if pressed to do so. Your senses are tuned, thrilled to be on a mission, knowing there is a smokey, tender treat if you achieve success. Those animals tasted delicious, and bonding with my host brothers in the adventures were some of my favorite memories of the entire summer. Bushmeat hunting and fishing have supported humans for millennia. With an overabundance of food available to anyone in modern, developed countries, hunting and fishing are largely recreational pastimes and not a necessity. However, in large swaths of poorer countries, bushmeat hunting is a critical source of nutrition, and fishing keeps hundreds of millions of families alive. As human beings have populated the world and grown in numbers, the effects of hunting wild populations of animals and fish for food have been staggering.

For millions of years, an abundance of megafauna, the large animals, was a prominent feature of the land and oceans. However, in the last 20,000 years, with the rise of human beings, something profound happened to Earth's ecology. In the blink of an eye in terms of the eons of their existence, megafauna have largely disappeared from vast portions of our planet. They have become actually or functionally extinct. For example, after human beings arrived and expanded about 12,000 years ago in the western hemisphere via the land bridge that existed between Asia and North America, nearly all the megafauna soon disappeared.[105] Prior to the arrival of humans, the western hemisphere harbored 27 species of megaherbivores heavier than 1,000 kg (2,200 lbs) that included remarkable creatures such as mastodons, mammoths, horses, camels, ox, and enormous ground sloths measuring to 6 m (20 ft) in length from head to tail. All are now extinct. Of 50 megaherbivore species that existed then across Earth, only nine remain today, which are five species of rhinoceros, three species of elephants, and the hippopotamus, with all of these survivors severely depleted in numbers and range. Of the species we lost, 10 were larger than the largest remaining terrestrial species on earth, the African bush elephant. Severe losses are also seen among large herbivores, especially in North America where 23 of 36 species have become extinct. Of the 13 species of megacarnivores present as humans arrived in the Americas, only four remain. We lost awe-inspiring predators like the saber-toothed tiger, American lion, American cheetah, giant short-faced bear, and dire wolf. Of the 15 megacarnivore species heavier than 100 kg (220 lbs) alive on the planet when humans began migrating globally, only six remain today. The predominant theory as to why these extinctions occurred is that humans were "superpredators" that were able to hunt even the largest mammals that had previously faced little predation pressure. Our ancestors killed off large numbers, perhaps down to the last individual for many species, and the populations of species with any remaining survivors were too small to produce enough offspring to maintain long-term sustainable populations. Extinctions, reductions in abundance, and local extirpations of wild megafauna have continued into recent times driven by habitat loss and direct consumption of those animals and their body parts. Today, it requires armed guards to protect many of these last mega-size species, and even with protection, poachers continue to erase them from our planet.

With the large, easy-to-find prey species hunted near or to extinction, people have moved on to smaller species, and the increased human population size has greatly magnified the effects of hunting wildlife to the point where terrestrial mammals are experiencing a massive collapse in their population sizes and geographical ranges around the world.[106] Bushmeat hunting for mostly food and medicinal products is the core driver in a global crisis causing over 300 terrestrial mammal species to be threatened with extinction. Poaching pressure is increasing in many parks and reserves as numbers in unprotected areas have drastically declined. Due to widespread overhunting, many wildlands have become "empty forests," devoid of nearly all animals that previously filled the green cathedrals of nature with their calls.[107] Ecologists can walk for days through remote wildlands and encounter or hear virtually no wildlife. No monkeys howling. No birds calling. Nearly everything that could be hunted for food has already been removed. This is done by local people to feed their families, but significant numbers are killed by commercial hunters that collect large numbers of animals and ship them to urban cities to be sold in bushmeat markets. In many cultures, eating bushmeat is considered a delicacy or sign of status.[108] Regions with the most species threatened by bushmeat hunting include Asia, especially southeast Asia, and Africa. Wild meat is an important food source for humans worldwide. For example, in the Brazilian Amazon, an estimated 89,000 tons of meat with a market value of approximately $200 million are harvested. Harvests of large mammals in the Congo basin of Africa are estimated to be five times higher than in the Brazilian Amazon.[106]

This widespread burden on ecosystems can have wide-ranging negative effects that cascade far beyond the loss of the hunted species. Their roles are crucial to ecosystem stability and their loss can result in rapid, widespread, and potentially irrevocable changes. Without large herbivore prey, predators will suffer and may not survive. Large predators and herbivores provide "top-down" control on ecosystems, which acts as a balancing effect on environmental, or "bottom-up" factors, such as primary productivity or climate. A classic example was the historic and near-complete removal of sea otters from the Pacific coast of North America.[109] Without these cunning mammals present, a favorite prey of theirs, sea urchins were released from predatory pressure and urchin populations exploded. Their massive numbers overwhelmed their food source, kelp. They chew through the base of the plant, clipping it off to float away and die. The urchins cut the forests into near oblivion. The kelp provided the primary productivity for the ecosystem, harvesting the sun's energy and producing the primary source of food that cascaded through the entire food web. Without otters, the towering, majestic kelp forests turned barren. The kelp made up the three-dimensional habitat, and disappearing along with it were all the other species that found refuge, food, and symbioses within it. A similar process occurs in forest ecosystems, often allowing small mammals to increase in population size, cascading into transformation of invertebrate and plant communities. For example, without large mammals, many species of trees lose their method of seed dispersal, affecting their long-term survival and forest structure.[110] Smaller mammals like monkeys and bats, which feed on fruits, are well documented as key to seed dispersal and forest structure.[111] In addition to being seed dispersers, bats are also critical specialized pollinators that are unlikely to be replaced.[112] Their extirpation can potentially end reproduction for many species of plants. Yet of mammals under 1 kilogram threatened by hunting, bats are the most affected group.[106] Eliminating large numbers of animals and species in an ecosystem radiates out, affecting everything else associated with it, including humans.

Bushmeat hunting is at the root of the Covid-19 epidemic.[1] It is not the first disease with dire consequences for humans coming from hunting and eating wild animals, and it will not be the last. About 60% of known infectious diseases and 75% of all new, emerging, or re-emerging diseases in humans have animal origins.[113] Seven types of coronaviruses are found in humans. All of them came from animals. Zoonotic disease transmission (from animals to humans) is a direct result of stalking, killing, transporting, and butchering wildlife for human consumption. This creates high levels of direct contact of body fluids that are thought to have been important in emergence of Ebola, HIV-1 and -2, anthrax, salmonellosis, simian foamy virus, SARS-CoV-1 (2003 SARS outbreak), and SARS-CoV-2 (Covid-19 pandemic). The latter is best hypothesized to have originated from horseshoe bats, *Rhinolophus*, and potentially transmitted directly to people or via an intermediate species such as pangolin. Both bats and pangolin are widely hunted and consumed in Asia. Pangolin are illegally trafficked more frequently and in greater numbers than almost any other species in the world. They are killed for the meat and scales, which are believed, incorrectly, to have medicinal properties, but also eaten as an exclusive delicacy. In 2003, SARS was spread to humans from bats via captured palm civets, a cute mammal that splatters its feces to mark territory – a habit that would readily spread disease in live animal markets. If people stopped eating wildlife, this disease emergence route would be dramatically reduced.[114] Bushmeat hunting can cause disease in humans not just from the direct interaction with the prey eaten, but via cascading effects on ecosystems. As large predators are removed from forests and other habitats, rodents are released from this predatory pressure, just as urchins were released from pressure from sea otters. Rodents are key vectors for carrying and transmitting disease, often through fleas that live upon them. Rodent-flea transmission was the underlying cause of the Black Death of the middle ages, the deadliest pandemic recorded in human history, which resulted in the deaths of up to 200 million people in Eurasia and North Africa. Experimental evidence has shown that in the absence of large wildlife, human disease-carrying rodent and flea populations can increase dramatically.[115]

Like overhunting on land, overfishing in our rivers, lakes, seas, and oceans is having global consequences that will affect entire ecosystems as well as human health and wellness. Only about half of the described freshwater fish species have been evaluated for their conservation status, and of these, 31% are threatened with extinction.[116] Like the largest species on land, freshwater mega-fishes, those heavier than 30 kg (66 lbs), have experienced a staggering global loss, with populations declining by 94%.[55] Although direct exploitation through fishing is important, many other factors also affect freshwater fish including pollution, habitat loss, climate change, and invasive species. In the marine environment, the principal threats are overfishing and habitat loss. More than half of North American marine fishes are threatened from overfishing and the majority of marine fish extinctions have been caused primarily by overfishing.[116] The average state of global fish stocks is poor and declining, and a business-as-usual scenario projects further continued collapse for many of the world's fisheries. The old black-and-white photos of marine giants caught 50-100 years ago hint at what we have lost, and data backs it up. Examining recreationally caught "trophy" reef fish with photographs taken in Key West, Florida, from 1956 to 2007 revealed an amazing 90% decline in weight.[54] A major shift in species composition occurred as well. Landings in the late 1950s were dominated by large groupers, sharks, and other large predatory fish, with an average length about the same as the height of an adult human. In stark contrast, landings in 2007 were mostly small snappers with an average length that would not even reach up to the height of your knee. Their size dropped 80% in just a few decades. The big fish are virtually gone from our global waters, and we are chewing our way progressively through the smaller ones.

A fishing practice that is truly devastating our oceans is trawling. Bottom trawls are used to catch fish, crustaceans, and bivalves living in, on, or above the seabed by dragging nets or dredges behind a ship along the seafloor. This activity, especially when repeated frequently in an area can have dramatic effect, with some forms of trawling removing 41% of all biomass with a single pass.[117] The gear dragged across ocean bottoms stirs up sediments, dramatically reduces biomass, and can completely obliterate ecosystems that took thousands of years to form. Video footage from research submersibles has shown areas that previously harbored a complex mix of sponges, corals, and other life forms being erased of these life forms with vast flattened plains of barren rubble left after trawling.[118] This would be the equivalent of driving a line of bulldozers through a forest, demolishing everything in their path, in order to uncover and capture a few species of animals like rabbits, squirrels, or deer that could be eaten. The rest of the biodiversity, including the trees that give the ecosystem structure, are destroyed, leaving lifeless wastelands. As nearshore continental shelf areas have been overfished, trawling has been progressing into deeper areas of the ocean, where life forms grow much slower, and destruction will last far longer. Trawling is a major threat to the deep seafloor ecosystem at a global scale, part of an international fishing fleet estimated to have over 3.7 million vessels, more than twice what existed in 1950. However, the amount of fish caught per unit of fishing effort, like the amount caught in a day of fishing, has declined by 80% since then.[119] This clearly shows the increasing pressure of fisheries on ocean resources, but unseen to most people's eyes is the massive scale of destruction that this fishing has caused, an obliteration of life hidden below the waves.

~ Grazing ~

Mankind has hunted, fished, and gathered for millions of years. A next step in our evolution toward food stability, a better guarantee of a ready source of on-hand nutrition, involved following, maintaining, and eating grazers on pastures. This pathway eventually took us toward livestock domestication as mankind progressively developed into more sedentary communities. Pastoral societies, which are typically nomadic, involve daily lives that are centered around following and tending of herds of wild or semi-wild animals including cattle, camels, sheep, goats, yaks, llamas, reindeer, and horses. Wild animals were progressively selected to benefit people. Some pastoral cultures still exist today and are typically found in more extreme environments and more marginal lands where poor soils, cold or hot temperatures, and lack of water make growing crops very difficult. These animals turn wild grasses that are inedible by humans into food – meat and milk – and other valuable products. Large grazers managed by pastoralists can be key top-down ecosystem maintaining species in grassland environments, as the buffalo were once on the North American plains. They help maintain healthy ecosystems and biodiversity in grasslands by preventing them from evolving into dense shrublands or forests, recycling nutrients, and helping maintain this habitat for many other grassland-occupying species. However, this beneficial ecological role is one that requires a delicate balance of eating just the right amount, and not too much more. Pastoralists traditionally followed herds as they naturally moved on after briefly grazing for a few days in a region, following the rains and ensuing photosynthesis to find greener pastures elsewhere. People left the grazed pasture to recover and regrow, perhaps not visiting again for a year or longer. This pattern is at the heart of a healthy grassland ecosystem, and it was an activity that worked well until human population increased and the numbers of grazing livestock increased with them. In many parts of the world, the rest and recovery cycle for the pasture was progressively eliminated. Today, much of the grazing in the world is continuous, where cattle and other livestock are fenced in, and forced to graze the same area in greatly reduced cycles of time.

Grazing systems cover about 40% of the global terrestrial ice-free land surface.[120] More than one-third of the land in the U.S. is used for livestock grazing – by far the largest land-use type in the contiguous 48 states.[121] Though well-managed systems do exist, overgrazing has become a plague, like locusts, on much of our planet's grasslands. This is altering the composition of the Earth's surface in profound ways that is not beneficial to livestock, wildlife, or humans. An easy-to-spot sign of overgrazing of grasslands is gully erosion, which occurs with the loss of groundcover. Without sufficient plant cover and root structure, rain no longer lands softly and soaks gently into the ground, but instead splashes and rushes across a hard surface, carrying the topsoil with it. Water follows the path of least resistance and soon finds itself combining into small streams that cut into the ground. Over time, these cuts grow in width and depth. They meet downstream, resulting in larger, more powerful flows that cut with more force into the earth. Although there are examples of ranchers in the western United States practicing more sustainable methods of rotational grazing that can regenerate soils, much of the land out west is widely scarred by extensive gully erosion from many decades of poor grazing management, some lingering from overgrazing that occurred over a century ago.[122] The ecological costs of livestock grazing are arguably stronger than that of any other western land use, destroying native vegetation, damaging soils and stream banks, and contaminating waterways with excessive sediments and fecal waste.[123] With a keen eye driving down any highway or rural road in our country, especially in rolling hills where grazing takes place, you can spot gully erosion scarring the landscape nearly everywhere you look. It is a sign that many other cascading effects are occurring within the ecosystem.

The soils that are eroded from overgrazed lands are washed downstream where they have dire consequences for freshwater and marine habitats. The suspended soils turn previously clear streams cloudy, blocking the light that drives primary productivity and also directly harming many organisms, including filter feeders like mussels, which are overwhelmed by the sediments. A screaming canary in the coal mine, no group of organisms in the U.S. is more threatened than freshwater mussels. About 70% are extinct, probably extinct, or in immediate threat of extinction.[124] Some of the most dramatic impacts grazing animals have on waterways occur as a result of the common practice of letting livestock have free access to enter streams and riparian habitat, the vegetation that grows along waterways. Livestock consume this vegetation, trample soils, erode streambanks, and can completely change the habitat into one of barren topsoil that easily erodes away. The removal and exclusion of cattle can result in dramatic changes in affected riparian vegetation, even without replanting or other active restoration efforts. Up to a 90% decrease in the amount of bare soil quickly occurs as grasses, willows, and other plants explode in growth with cattle exclusion.[123] The loss of grassland habitat and soil erosion from overgrazing also help drive climate change. Native, high-diversity grasslands are important for extracting and storing carbon from the atmosphere, sequestering it in the soils that these ecosystems build below their extensive and deep-penetrating root networks.[125] Remove the vegetation, expose the soil to erosion, and the carbon is released. The mechanism for storing the carbon is wrecked by overgrazing.

Like many types of environmental damage, overgrazing is driven by profits. However, the damage from grazing is subsidized by all of us. Livestock grazing is ubiquitous in the western United States, comprising nearly a third of the area of the lower 48 states. It is promoted, protected, and subsidized with hundreds of millions of dollars by federal agencies on approximately 270 million acres of public land in the 11 western states. That means you as a taxpayer are giving your tax money to people to graze on your land. They earn profits, subsidized by you, to create heart disease, and our commonly owned land is degraded and eroded. This history of subsidized government support is centuries old. Keystone predators like the grizzly and Mexican gray wolf were driven extinct in the southwestern U.S. by government-sponsored "predator control" programs designed to support the livestock industry. Without your tax support, the grazing industry would have a tough time surviving, but for now, you are helping pay for their profits whether you buy their meat or not. In 2014, resource economists commissioned by the Center for Biological Diversity found that money the federal government earned from grazing fees on public lands was $125 million less than what the federal government spent on the program.[126] They also found that federal grazing fees are 93% less than fees charged for similar private grazing land. At only $1.69 per animal per month for each cow and calf that grazes the public land, the deal for ranchers is incredible. Wouldn't it be nice if it cost you less than $2 a month to feed your dog or cat, letting U.S. taxpayers pick up the rest of the bill? Given the massive damage grazing does to much of the dry western states, it is even more stunning that western federal rangelands account for less than 3% of all forage fed to livestock in the United States.[126] If those rangelands were left alone, people who eat beef would hardly notice. Of course, ranchers who line their pockets with your money would notice. I have no doubt most ranchers are good, hardworking people trying to make a living, but the industry and the products they produce have serious negative effects on our lives.

The long-term effects of overgrazing on ecosystems and human society are exemplified in the place where mankind has been living in settled agricultural societies the longest – the Middle East. We all learned about the Fertile Crescent early in our schooling. It's the magical place where the Tigris and Euphrates Rivers meet, the lands where settled human agriculture and cultures first organized, forged metals, and eventually spread out and conquered the entire planet. The region has undergone the pressures of livestock grazing for about 11,000 years, and evidence indicates increasing pressures of grazing for over 5,000 years has caused much of its fertile lands to turn into deserts.[127] Today, the most common generalist grazers in the region are goats, often seen on their hind legs reaching up to nip at leaves as the lower vegetation has already been chewed into rocky barrens. To me, the sight of these goat herds on barren lands is the sign that the life of an ecosystem is being eaten "down to its bones." They are the last grazers, feeding on the remnants of what was historically vast valleys and hills that would come alive with diverse plant life after rains. The dire consequences of the rapid expansion of livestock that accompanied human population growth in the region have been realized by science for over a half century. It was estimated back in the 1960s that the number of range animals in Iran was 12 times the grazing capacity of the country. In central Turkey, it was estimated that over 90% of the livestock should be excluded from studied rangelands in order to avoid further damage.[128] However, warnings like those have rarely been heeded, and much of the Middle East has seen expanding deserts overtaking millions upon millions of acres where grasslands and forests once thrived. Combined with climate change, the consequences for humans are explosive.

It seems improbable that a war that has killed more than an estimated 200,000 people, leveled entire cities, drove an exodus of millions of people, involved many of the world's greatest military powers, and detonated hundreds of millions of dollars' worth of advanced weaponry including chemical weapons, cluster bombs, thermobaric weapons, and ballistic missiles could be caused by something as seemingly benign as sheep. We count them in our heads to coax our minds to sleep. Yet sheep, goats, and other livestock have ravaged the life-giving soils of the Syrian grasslands with dire consequences. Among the root causes of the ongoing Syrian War, which started nearly a decade ago, are overgrazing and desertification that has been an unfolding ecological disaster for more than half a century.[129]

In the 1970s, international aid organizations warned about ongoing overgrazing of the country's steppe, the dry grasslands that made up half of the country's area. Contiguous with grasslands in Iraq, Saudi Arabia, and Jordan, the area had been sustainably grazed via resting periods by pastoralists, the Bedouins, for many centuries. However, by the early 1960s, the government nationalized the steppe and investors increased stocking on the grasslands, greatly reducing the traditional resting phase that kept these ecosystems healthy. Overgrazing, loss of vegetation, and erosion quickly followed, driven by hungry Syrians growing from 4 million in the 1950s to 22 million in recent years. This vegetation previously helped slow rainfall runoff, infiltrating it into the ground where it built over centuries into aquifers. As grazing pressure increased, other agricultural crop production in the steppe east of the Euphrates also increased. Food crops and water-intensive crops like cotton expanded, irrigated by groundwater drawn up against the pull of gravity with fossil-fuel-powered pumps. Each year aquifer levels dropped. The wells were drilled deeper, many illegally.

A drought from 2006-2010, likely exacerbated by climate change that has made the region about 10% drier, combined with a sudden halt of government subsidies and ensuing soaring prices of fuel for wells, led to a rural agricultural catastrophe.[130] In the northeast, overgrazed lands could no longer support livestock and the industry was practically wiped out. Cereal prices doubled. Syria, for the first time in its history, was no longer self-reliant for food, but instead required massive international emergency food aid. A perfect storm of overgrazing, over-extraction of water, reliance on fossil fuels for food production, and background climate change coalesced and ignited. Malnutrition took off. Millions of refugees were displaced to urban areas. War soon broke out, a catastrophe exacerbated by the cruelties of a military dictatorship. The effects are ongoing and will be felt long into the future by Syria and the entire world. Unfortunately, this perfect storm threatens to rise again in other lands where population growth, increasingly unsustainable food consumption and production patterns, and competing water demands collide under climate change.

~ Pasture Creation ~

As demand for beef expanded around the world, it became lucrative to create more pasture to support more cattle. Vast swaths of our planet have been deforested, and most of that deforested land has been converted to cattle pasture. The great forests of the eastern United States were felled for lumber and replaced with crops and beef and dairy cattle long ago, reaching their lowest extent of coverage in 1920. As the forests were cut, which removed vast interwoven networks of roots, the soils quickly eroded. Between the late 1800s and early 1900s, settlers in the eastern United States caused extensive soil erosion that would have taken thousands of years to occur under natural rates. So much soil was washed into rivers that their flows could only carry away less than 10% of this eroded soil.[131] The rest was deposited in the river valleys. Their waters will likely be laden with excess sediment for many decades to come, and any efforts to restore these habitats will affect ecosystems further downstream as this legacy sediment would be stirred up. Although deforestation to create grazing lands for livestock in the United States, Europe, and the rest of the temperate regions affected ecosystems extensively around the northern hemisphere and created long-term problems, what is ongoing in the southern hemisphere is of critical importance now.

The biodiverse tropical forest-endowed countries, like Costa Rica, have little natural pasture. They developed new lands for grazing livestock by destroying forests, removing lumber trees, and typically burning away the remaining vegetation. Costa Rica cleared well over half of its forests for cattle, and this was replicated throughout much of Central America, often to supply North America with cheap beef. Many of those fast-food burgers I enjoyed as a child in the 1970s were devoured, unknowingly by myself, my family, or most Americans, at the expense of these forest ecosystems. By an overwhelming margin, the forests of the Amazon basin have been cleared to make way for cattle. That newly cleared, cow-dung-filled pasture that I picked mushrooms from in 1989 in Colombia has been replicated thousands upon thousands of times across many countries, causing continuous additive degradation.

When a tropical forest is cleared for pasture, the ecological effects are immediate and profound. Thousands of species of plants and animals can occupy just one acre of this habitat, no doubt including many species that are still unknown to science. In days, they can all be eliminated, cut, and scorched to the ground. Rare species that occupy small areas disappear without ever being discovered. Populations of more widespread species decrease as their habitat is gradually eliminated with ongoing clearing. Remaining forests progressively become smaller and smaller islands in a sea of pasture. These habitat islands are too small to support viable populations of many species and the clearings between them are like moats across which many species cannot cross. It may take many decades for the effects to fully manifest as populations gradually dwindle away within these remaining lifeboats. The pastures that replace these forests are biological wastelands in comparison to what was thriving there before the chainsaws and fire.

It may seem that the destruction of the myriad of species living in a tropical forest would be in itself the entire injury of creating cattle pasture upon its ground, but the damage cascades on. Just as occurred in the eastern United States, when forests are cleared in the tropics, erosion follows. However, in the tropics, where rainfall can be 10 times higher, the erosion of soils can be tremendous. This erosion effect has only grown stronger over time as the areas where forests in many countries are now cut have shifted. Much of the forest in lowland flat areas was cleared in years past, as it was much easier and cheaper to develop into agriculture. This is reflected in Costa Rica and many other tropical countries by the location of their national parks. They are predominantly situated in the mountains, as the flat lowlands were cut and developed before protecting ecosystems became politically important. As forest clearing for pasture migrates up into hills and mountains, gravity and the power it gives to flowing water magnifies erosion. The very shallow layer of topsoil can be stripped away in a single downpour. Relentless rains will continue to eat away into the earth, and even as grasses take hold following forest clearing, gully erosion is widespread and never ceasing.

Following deforestation and subsequent sedimentation, nearby freshwater tropical streams also experience a reduction in biodiversity. During the rainy season, rivers become choked with sediment, which is carried to the ocean. It then spreads with currents along coastlines. Seen from above, it looks like chocolate milk swirling and blending into the vibrant aqua blue of tropical seas. In other places it flows rust-red due to the high iron-oxide content of nutrient-poor tropical soils. Madagascar, the island nation located just off eastern Africa, has been severely battered by deforestation. When viewed from outer space, it looks like it is bleeding to death as red waters flow out of all its river mouths. Madagascar is a unique country extremely high in endemic species, including 84% of its vertebrates, meaning they are found nowhere else.[132] The country and its signature endemic species, lemurs, inspired the creation of a DreamWorks animated film franchise, featuring widely recognized voices of stars for the lovable characters. It has grossed over a 2 billion dollars in global sales.[133] I would bet that virtually no one who has laughed with their children during those funny movies has any idea that the life-giving soil of the real Madagascar is washing away day by day into the ocean. The bleeding of that nation is caused primarily by clearing forests for livestock, which now cover half of the country's land. Along with the death of those forests was the extensive disappearance of lemurs. Out of 111 known species of lemurs, 105 have been evaluated as critically endangered, endangered, or vulnerable, making 95% of the lemur population at high risk of extinction. This is the highest percentage of threatened members of any large group of mammals or any large group of vertebrates on Earth.[134] Ironically, McDonald's licensed and gave away *Madagascar* movie-character toys in Happy Meal promotions – a toy lemur with your kid's burger to commemorate the ultimate cow-driven cause of the furry creature's pending extinction.

Along coastlines, the sediment-laden water from deforestation and overgrazed pasture blocks sunlight, decreasing primary productivity of life below. It also gradually settles out, pulled to the bottom. However, on the seafloor lining the coasts of many tropical countries and islands are ecosystems with biodiversity and services just as critical as tropical forests: coral reefs. The increased turbidity of the water decreases the sunlight corals require, and the settling sediment smothers corals and leads to substantial mortality. This has been documented in reefs around the world, including those in Madagascar.[135] In addition to sedimentation from forest clearing, tropical reefs are also threatened by overfishing. Equally, climate change is a growing threat to reefs as increasing greenhouse gases drive warmer atmospheric and ocean temperatures. Higher water temperatures around reefs cause coral bleaching, where corals under heat stress expel the symbiotic algae that provide them with energy and imbue them with color. Under long and repeated heat stress events, the loss of the algae causes widespread death and loss of coral cover. Higher atmospheric concentrations of carbon dioxide (CO_2), one of the gases causing climate change, also diffuse into our oceans, causing higher CO_2 concentrations in seawater. This dissolved CO_2 makes the ocean more acidic, which counteracts the chemical process that corals employ to build their calcium-carbonate skeletons. Already shown to be affecting reefs, as CO_2 levels continue to rise, ocean acidity levels and their destructive force will increase as well.[136] Clearing forests for pasture directly releases tremendous amounts of carbon, which was locked up in the vegetation and soils, into the atmosphere. The cattle that replace the diverse forest ecosystem burp copious amounts of methane, which is roughly 30 times more potent as a heat-trapping gas in the atmosphere than CO_2.

Choosing to eat a burger or steak that was raised on pasture carved out of forests, especially tropical forests, is tied intimately into a diverse web of effects that radiate out and diminish life on Earth, including human life. Choosing beef means choosing these effects. Burger King, McDonald's, and many other retailers around the world still buy Brazilian beef or feed crops that were born out destruction of the forests of the Amazon or adjacent Cerrado.[137] It is served up on plates around the world, with leading importers including Russia, China, Italy, and Germany. Brazil is the leading exporter of beef, comprising 20% of global beef exports.[82] Imports from Brazil into the United States, the largest consumer of beef in the world, have just been again approved after several years of bans due to quality control issues including blood clots, bone, and other materials in Brazilian beef.[138] When meat processing plants in the U.S. slowed production during Covid-19, Nicaragua, the northern and equally biodiverse neighbor of Costa Rica, became the third largest supplier of frozen beef imports to the U.S., reaching an all-time high for the nation. This increased demand then drove demand for more land by ranchers, some who are using fear and murder to intimidate indigenous communities into giving up their land to cows. Armed cattle ranchers have attacked indigenous people, burning homes and killing at least 10 people to date, including shooting a 14-year-old girl, in order to steal land.[139] Brazilian, Nicaraguan, or any imported beef can be labeled "Product of the USA" as long as it is processed in some way in the United States, including simply cutting large pieces of beef into smaller ones. If you eat beef anywhere on our planet, a strong chance exists that it comes to you via destruction of tropical forests, which also leads to catastrophic consequences for local indigenous people. This includes the largest tropical forest ecosystem on Earth, the Amazon, and its adjacent southern neighbor, the drier savannah-forest system of the Cerrado, which is considered one of the most endangered ecosystems on the planet.

~ Monoculture Feed Crop Cultivation ~

Though enormous portions of our forests have been razed and replaced with pasture for livestock, increasingly they are being cleared to plant feed crops, the most important being soy.

As nutrition-packed as soybeans are, only a trickle of the world's production is consumed directly by people. Most is fed as protein-dense soybean meal to livestock after the oil has been extracted as an ingredient to be used in a wide swath of processed foods and other products. Soybeans and soybean meal are shipped around the world to supply CAFOs that raise cattle, pigs, chickens, and fish. Most of these soy products come from Brazil, the world's top soy exporter, grown on land once covered by forests in the Amazon and Cerrado. Over 80% of agricultural land in the Cerrado is soy production, covering an area about the size of Missouri. In just one year from August 2018 to July 2019, an area equivalent to 1.2 million football fields of natural Cerrado vegetation was cleared.[140] This paralleled a 30% increase in deforestation in the Amazon in 2018. Beef cattle and soy production are the primary proximate causes of current and past deforestation in the Amazon and the Cerrado. Demand for meat from people all over the world is the ultimate cause. If you eat beef, pork, or chicken nearly anywhere in the world, it is likely that some of the soy that fattened it came from Brazil. The Cerrado still has 23 million hectares of open land that could be converted to soy. That will only happen with continuing demand for meat. The choice to reduce that demand is ours.

People in the United States may contend that they only eat 100% American beef or that our American livestock production systems don't destroy rainforests. They may believe that their choices are not harming the environment. As discussed previously regarding livestock grazing, we have already greatly altered grasslands and forests, lost massive amounts of their soils that took thousands of years to create, and altered downstream freshwater ecosystems that are today among the most endangered habitats in our nation. All that degradation to produce a small sliver of the beef that is consumed here. The production of feed crops in the U.S. is equally if not more devastating and wasteful. After Brazil, the United States is the world's second largest exporter of beef and soy products, which are also shipped to CAFOs around the planet.[82] The Midwest, at the heart of our nation, has often and warmly been referred to as the "bread basket of America." The life source of our nation. We imagine a cornucopia of baked goods spilling out from its waving fields of grains, consumed by healthy, hungry, hardworking people. Breakfast cereals. Warm breads. Crunchy snacks. That image, however, is vastly different from reality. The heartland of America would be more accurately referred to as our meat basket – a use very bad for our hearts.

About one-third of the cropland in the United States is used to grow feed crops for livestock. Corn is by far the most widely grown crop in the United States, covering the equivalent of about 69 million football fields in 2019. If it were confined to a state, it would just about fill Montana. If it was all laid out in a square, it would take you six hours to drive across it. About 40% of the crop is fed to livestock as a carbohydrate source, supplemented with soy as a protein source. The next largest use of the corn crop is to produce ethanol fuel, and the rest is used in over 4,000 other products or exported.[141] Soybean acreage is just about equivalent to corn. Over 70% of the soybeans grown in the United States are used for animal feed, with poultry as the leading consumer, followed by hogs, dairy, beef, and aquaculture. In 2018, the top six largest sources of income from the sale of U.S.-produced farm commodities were all animal products or feed for them – cattle, corn, soybeans, dairy products, chickens, and hogs.[142] Like Costa Rica, the largest use of all land in the United States is for livestock. Between pastures and cropland used to produce feed, 41% of all the land in the contiguous states is used by us for livestock production.[121] The amount we use for crops we directly eat is only 4%. As that rule in ecology predicts, we roughly use 10 times as much land to feed our livestock than the land we use to grow plant foods to directly feed ourselves.

The destruction of our country's land, soils, waters, and the money generated from it by animal products is something I only began to understand much later in adulthood. Ironically, my favorite memories of childhood were actively intertwined with clearing forests, fostering erosion, and degradation of waterways to feed livestock. As a young boy, the person I looked up to the most was my grandfather, John Kenner. He was quiet, patient, methodical, and he wasted nothing. A plumber by trade, he was self-industrious like many a man living through and losing his money in the Great Depression. He built his own home and small vacation cottage on a lake. To a kid, however, the trait that intrigued me most was his unspoken reverence for the peace and respite of nature, and his joy in revealing to Brett and me the beauty of life and its creatures. He was calm, cool, and comfortable in nature. During summers, my family spent a week at the cottage along with my grandparents, aunts, uncles, and cousins. The kids swam, chased lightning bugs, and spent entire days searching for clams, frogs, turtles, and snakes. We would shadow Gramps when he came back from a morning of fishing on the lake, learning how to clean a bass, our eyes wide open as the inner workings of the creatures were dissected and described. During a long pause between two sentences, Gramps would often purse his lips and spit out a big splat of tobacco on the ground. With a sly look, he would say it attracted the fish when he spit in the lake. When he opened up the crinkled envelope-package of Mail Pouch Tobacco to take out a fresh wad, he would angle the opening toward us in offering. I loved the sweet, musty fermented odor. It's honied smell seemed like it would taste delicious, but just one pinch was enough for me to learn smells can be very deceiving. The acrid, bitter, burning leaves made me expel it immediately, coughing, followed by spitting out the lingering stain on my taste buds. Gramps chuckled, knowing we would never try it again.

Around Easter and Thanksgiving, our family would make the journey from Cleveland's suburbs, headed west to the edge of the state. I always anticipated those journeys because it meant exploring the woods with Gramps. My grandparents lived in a very small Midwestern farming town, Hicksville, Ohio. Visiting with my cousins was fun, but the real adventure was with Gramps, who was sure to take us out to the 80 acres of land he owned a 10-minute drive down a roller-coaster hilly road into the countryside. It was always the highlight of our visit. On the drive out, we often had to slow down to pass the shiny black horse-drawn buggies of the Amish with caution. But on a clear straightaway, he put the pedal to the floor, driving much faster than my father ever did. Our stomachs would drop with exciting yelps as we crested the biggest hills. For a moment, a grin would slightly break his usual stoic look. At the time, those 80 acres were my favorite place on earth. The "front 40" was farmland that sloped down to the back half, which was the deep shady woods crossed with a meandering stream.

Gramps always took us on a stroll through the woods, an intentionally quiet walk except for the occasional farts he would rumble out of his gray pants or the splat of tobacco in the soil. He gathered edible mushrooms to be his treat later and wild apples for our immediate pleasure. The cool, tart crisp of a wild apple with leaves crunching under foot is indelible in my mind. He always made sure to take us by the mound of earth that was peppered with holes where groundhogs and fox liked to den. Peering into those depths, I often tossed an apple core as an offering that I hoped might lead to a glimpse of fur, always to no avail. After an hour or so of exploring, Gramps usually put us to work, which meant improving conditions for the front 40 acres. That acreage rotated between feed corn and soy, but by our visit in fall it was wide-open muddy rows covered in the rough stubble of brown cornstalks remaining long past the harvest. We sometimes helped Gramps clearing the edge of the forest back, making a little more room for crops to be planted the next year. He would cut the trees for wood with a chainsaw, and we would help burn the remaining trimmings that were left. Great bonfires of brush would dance and mesmerize, and we would toss branches into the roaring orange glow. The power of fire intimidated, and revealed its power to erase when my dangling Bugs Bunny mitten hooked unknowingly onto a branch I threw and leapt with it into the inferno. That carrot-chomping, buck-toothed grin melted and burst into flames, sent swirling into the sky along with all that carbon dioxide.

We also walked the fields checking on the terra-cotta drainage piping Gramps had been laying down for years, improving the fields to combat flooding that often plagued the clay-rich soils. The drain pipes were oriented to shunt water out of the field and into the creek. After scanning the hand-dug ditches being laid with pipe, we ended up at the creek, which was my favorite place. We walked the bank, and Brett and I would scamper in and drag out branches that gathered leaves and debris, freeing up the creek to flow faster. The goal was to make sure the corn and soybean fields would drain quickly, unbound by the meanderings of an unmanaged forest creek. When it did rain, that creek turned from a clear bubbling stream into a churning, racing torrent of brown. Little by little, the soil that covered the front 40 washed away into that creek, as it was doing in millions of creeks across our nation. Corn and soy fields are highly susceptible to erosion, and walking through one will always reveal gully erosion snaking across their surface. The fields are plowed, turning and loosening up soil. Lack of any vegetation early in the spring before planting and later in the fall after harvest left the soils exposed to wind and rain. Consistent and often heavy rains are common in spring and fall. Even during the full crop cover of later summer, soils are still susceptible to erosion. Over time, annual erosion adds up.

Like Ohio, Iowa is corn and soy country, with fields covering about two-thirds of the state. Iowa is blessed with some of the richest soils in our nation and the entire world, developed over thousands of years under prairie plants that were held tightly by their roots. When Americans started farming that heartland state, the topsoil was on average about 14-16 inches deep. Today it is 6-8 inches deep.[143] About half of all the rich, priceless topsoil that took nature great lengths of patient time to slowly create in Iowa has eroded away. It is a resource overwhelmingly mined and washed down the drain to make meat. Combined across the meat basket farms of America, the loss of soil is stunning. Washing off the farms and fields within the Mississippi watershed, spilling into the great freshwater artery that drains 40% of the area of the lower 48 states, is the soil that gives us life – literally the food on our tables. Each year, the equivalent of nearly 400 million pickup-truck loads of soil washes out the mouth of the Mississippi watershed into the Gulf of Mexico. Each decade the amount of this rich soil could fill the Superdome stadium in New

Orleans more than 500 times as it passes nearby on its way to the ocean.[144] It washes out decade after decade. It is gone forever.

Carried along with that soil are the fossil-fuel-based chemicals that fertilize the fields, eliminate weeds, and kill pests. Making the fertilizers, herbicides, and pesticides that we apply to agriculture requires energy, and the processes release greenhouse gases. The three main components of fertilizer are the elements nitrogen, phosphorus, and potassium, referred to collectively as NPK. These nutrients are required by life. Phosphorus is a component of cell membranes and nucleic acids, which form the backbone of DNA. Nitrogen is a key part of amino acids, which make up proteins that are the machinery of life. We nor any other life would exist without phosphorus or nitrogen. Our atmosphere is rich in nitrogen gas, N_2, but in order for life to use it, this gas first needs to be converted into a form that plants can use. Legumes, including soy, can fix nitrogen gas directly from the atmosphere. Through a partnership with bacteria located in specialized structures on their roots, legumes can extract nitrogen gas and incorporate it into their tissues. However, most plants, including corn, need a non-gaseous supply of nitrogen in solid forms of nitrate, nitrite, or ammonia present in the soil that their roots can absorb. In nature and organic agriculture, this comes from other decomposing organisms or manure – natural soil building. However, in most agricultural fields, including those growing feed crops, that nitrogen comes in the form of fertilizer that is produced from fossil fuels. In fertilizer production, the nitrogen is extracted from air and combined with hydrogen, typically extracted from methane in natural gas, to make ammonia. This reaction, called the Haber-Bosch process, is performed at temperatures around $500°C$ and at pressures 60-180 times higher than atmospheric pressure.[145] This requires large amounts of energy, which means burning fossil fuels and CO_2 release. For every ammonia molecule generated, the process releases one molecule of carbon dioxide as a coproduct. Those ammonia molecules that become fertilizers then transform into proteins in crops, livestock, and then us.

We are literally constructed from the hydrogen in natural gas, extracted by drilling and fracking it from the ground, which has many negative environmental consequences. That hydrogen most likely passed through corn and livestock before it became you. However, of all the nitrogen that is created to sustain food production, less than 10% actually enters human mouths. The rest is lost to the environment.[146] Around 40% of total commercially applied NPK is put on corn, and 10% on soybeans.[147] Half of the fertilizer we generate is applied on the two crops that drive our animal product and junk food industries. Unfortunately, not all of that fertilizer makes it into the crops. Intimately linked to soil erosion is the runoff of nutrients from fertilizer. In high-erosion corn fields, more than two-thirds of the nitrogen and phosphorous applied can run off along with soil into waterways.[148] On farms with better erosion controls, runoff can be far less, but nitrogen can also percolate down through soil into water tables and migrate underground into waterways. The tile drainage pipes used on my grandfather's farm are also used on about half of the other farms in Ohio, which provides a rapid route for delivering soil and fertilizer runoff into waterways. That stream that I loved exploring and clearing of debris for Gramps carries on. It is drawn by gravity, merges with other streams, joins the Maumee River, and eventually empties into the far western edge of Lake Erie. The fertilizer from that farm, combined with thousands of other farms throughout the region, flowed year upon year into the lake.

Just as top-down controls, like sea otters or other carnivores, are key in an ecosystem, altering bottom-up controls can produce equally profound radiating effects. A key bottom-up control in any ecosystem is the amount of nutrients available as they alter the type and magnitude of primary productivity. Shifting the amount and proportion of nutrients can send the entire ecosystem out of balance. Adding nutrients to a freshwater lake causes algae suspended in the water column to thrive and multiply into blooms. Those blooms block light reaching the lake bottom, shading out plants. As the algae dies, it is consumed by bacteria, whose metabolism uses up the oxygen in the water, making it uninhabitable for other organisms, including fish, which require dissolved oxygen to survive. This dead zone ebbs and recedes with the seasons as water, excessive nutrients, and sunshine interact. More nutrients and sunshine create more algae, more bacteria, and less oxygen. Western Lake Erie is now plagued by harmful algae blooms. The dominant species of algae in the bloom, *Microcystis*, produces the toxin microcystin, which can cause numbness, dizziness, vomiting, and liver damage – dangerous to people and animals. The 2014 algae bloom caused 400,000 residents of Toledo, Ohio to go without drinking water from their taps for three days and in 2019 it covered 620 square miles.[149] Water bodies across our nation and the world are increasingly plagued by algal blooms and dead zones, driven primarily by fertilizers applied to feed crops. The mouth of the Mississippi River, where those millions of loads of topsoil are washed out, has a dead zone that can cover up to 7,000 square miles, fed by over 3 billion pounds of nitrogen and 300 million pounds of phosphorus carried with that soil from farms each year.[144]

Excess nutrients can affect ecosystems and economies far from the fields upon which they are placed. In the warm subtropical waters off Miami, the ocean surface is increasingly being filled with a species of brown floating algae, *Sargassum*. Anyone who has walked the beaches of Florida or the Caribbean has come across it, washed up along the shore. It forms a small branching bunch, outfitted with little gas-filled floats that keep it on the surface. These individual bunches, pushed by wind and currents, gather together in floating mats. Living among and around these floating ecosystems are a myriad of life forms. Crabs and shrimp with colors and shapes to perfectly mimic the algae – an evolutionary camouflage – makes predation by young sea turtles and mahi-mahi more challenging. Sargassum mats are a favorite destination of sport fishermen and are a magical place to explore as a free diver, slipping under the mat to gaze up at a golden sunlit raft of life undulating above. Far out in the Atlantic Ocean, sargassum gathers in the center of a gyre, where the winds calm. Sailors for centuries have referred to this as the

Sargasso Sea, passing through it on their way between the old and new world. It was first reported by Christopher Columbus in the 15th century.

Since a tipping point in 2011, the annual aerial coverage of sargassum in the Atlantic has exploded to massive proportions. July sees a peak of sargassum growth, and during that month in 2018 it grew into a continuous belt reaching from Africa through all the Caribbean islands and up into the Gulf of Mexico to the outflow of the Mississippi — now called the Great Atlantic Sargassum Belt. Average monthly amounts of sargassum in the Atlantic were 10 times greater in 2018 than 2011.[150] Floating masses of seaweed are now piling up along the shores of southern Florida and the Caribbean to the great detriment of beach goers, boat owners, and the entire tourism industry. Living upon the sargassum are hydroids, relatives of jellyfish and anemones. Their branching tentacles are armed with harpoon-like stinging cells that inject enzymes into small prey that come within reach. Many people are also sensitive to those stinging cells, which induce pain, itching, redness, and swelling. After so much time in the ocean here in Miami, I have become highly sensitive. Brushing up against a bunch of sargassum with hydroids can leave me scratching with welts for days. A beach where the water surface now commonly looks like a minefield of sargassum keeps me on the sand. It will increasingly keep people from even wanting to visit the beach or the cities or countries where sand and surf have been the main draw and economic base. The sargassum comes in such relentless amounts that it builds up on the beach, reaching far up from the water's edge. It has accumulated as rows hundreds of yards long and 6 feet high. In the hot humid climate, it rapidly decays, releasing sulfur compounds with a foul, decaying-fish odor that is a perfect repellent for people. African coastlines are also being inundated, and Mexico even deployed its Navy to combat the invasion.

Here in Miami, the sargassum also works its way into Biscayne Bay, which lies between the mainland and the beaches. The floating clumps collect along the shallows and can extend 50 yards from shore, blocking light from reaching the bottom of the bay. This kills off the seagrass on the bottom, and a mixture of fetid decaying sargassum and other marine life turns the surface rancid with death and stench in the Miami heat. The summer days I used to spend exploring a crystal-clear bay with mask and snorkel are long gone. Today, dodging floating sargassum can at times make it unbearable. It feels like a final straw after witnessing the loss of most of the seagrass that covered the bottom only a decade ago, and all the amazing marine life that disappeared with it. The floating sargassum is also a hindrance for boats whose coolant intakes are commonly blocked from the bunches that get sucked in. Cities and countries reliant on oceanfront tourism are spending millions of dollars raking, burying, and removing sargassum to clear beaches for tourists. As soon as a beach is cleared, another wave appears, undermining all that effort. Today there are annual sargassum reinforcements stretching across the entire Atlantic, and the problem is on a strong trajectory to only get worse every year.

What is causing this invasion? A bottom-up ecosystem shift at the scale of an ocean. When one of the largest ecosystems on the planet is altered, the cascading effects can be profound and affect other equally massive ecosystems, with many effects unforeseen. As the Amazon is increasingly cleared, we can anticipate great changes to our planet and our lives as it is intimately interconnected to systems around the planet. It is a system so large and powerful that it drives rainfall patterns for an entire continent and it is central to regulating our global life support systems. The tip of an iceberg of change from our meddling with it is just coming into view. It is already revealing surprises, sargassum being an early warning. I am quite certain that no president, governor, hotel owner, or boater living within the warm waters that the Caribbean touches foresaw the effects on their lives, but what we all choose to eat can have huge ramifications. It will continue coming in brown stinging, stinking waves onto their shores. We are fertilizing the Atlantic Ocean and the sargassum is responding as plants do. The nutrients feeding all that algae are flowing out of the mouth of the Amazon.[150] Along with soils, it washes off the expanding fields of crops of the Amazon basin – crops grown overwhelmingly to make meat for people all around the world.

As detrimental as the nutrients in fertilizers can be to downstream ecosystems, we are also adding in a chemical soup of pesticides – herbicides, insecticides, and fungicides – that run off fields. As you could probably anticipate by now, corn uses more pesticide than any other crop, about 40% of all pesticides used in the United States. Soybeans rank second at about 20%.[151] Glyphosate, also known by the brand name Roundup, is the most widely used herbicide in the United States and the world, and the two crops to which it is applied the most are corn and soybeans. Most of the corn and soy grown in the United States are Roundup Ready crops, which means they have been genetically modified to tolerate glyphosate, which will kill other "pest" plants around them, thereby reducing competition from those plants for light, water, and nutrients.

Glyphosate and the commercial mixes of chemicals in which it is applied can be toxic to non-target plants, including downstream aquatic plants and algae, and other organisms like fish and amphibians. Glyphosate affects non-target organisms and water quality, modifying the structure and functionality of freshwater ecosystems.[152] The effects on one species can radiate out further, affecting humans. For example, since tadpoles of frogs are key organisms that eat and help control mosquito numbers, fewer of these amphibians can lead to more mosquitoes and greater exposure for us to mosquito-borne diseases like dengue fever.[153] The effects of this herbicide's toxicity on natural plant communities alters the ecology of systems exposed to it. Research has shown that applying glyphosate affects many non-target plants and can cause nearby plant diversity to decrease, even leading to the local extinction of native species.[154] As plant diversity decreases, the diversity of other animals utilizing these areas as habitat will also decrease.[155] Significant loss of biodiversity – up to 40% decrease for algae – has been shown to occur in freshwater communities contaminated with glyphosate.[156] High plant diversity is needed to maintain ecosystem services, especially in a changing world.[157]

The expansion of corn and soy throughout the United States into areas that harbored diverse wild flowering plants, maximizing the area planted on farms to increase income – combined with the growth of glyphosate use to control weeds on farmlands, roadsides, and other areas – has been implicated, along with other pesticides, in the massive decline of insects. A recent study in Germany documented an 80% reduction in biomass of flying insects in protected areas in just 27 years (1989–2016), likely due to surrounding agricultural intensification and its pesticide usage, year-round tillage, and increased use of fertilizers.[158] Without widespread weeds and wildflowers, insects lose the primary productivity upon which they feed. When I was a child in the 1970s, a summer road trip was marked by the windshield and front end of the family car plastered with hundreds of smooshed insects. Brett and I used to excitedly survey the plunder and gather butterflies, dragonflies, and other winged aliens from the radiator behind the grill. The loss of insects is likely a key link in the national decline of bird numbers. Since 1970, bird populations have dropped by nearly 3 billion across North America – an overall decline of 29%.[159] Monsanto developed and patented glyphosate as a weed killer in the early 1970s, first brought it to market in 1974, and then its use skyrocketed in the 1990s. Over two-thirds of the total amount applied has occurred in the past 10 years. Not enough research has been performed to show causal links, but widely broadcasting a chemical, in greater amounts than any pesticide in history, to kill plants that feed insects that feed birds, certainly deserves more attention and caution. Germany has called for glyphosate to be banned by the end of 2023 when the EU's current approval period for it expires because it wipes out insect populations crucial for ecosystems and pollination of food crops.[160]

As much as the application and runoff of glyphosate is detrimental to wildlife and ecosystems, the production of glyphosate is also directly linked with seriously harmful environmental problems. The elemental phosphorus used in its production comes from mines owned and operated by

Monsanto since the 1950s in Southeast Idaho near the town of Soda Springs, a small community of about 3,000 people. I've driven past the facilities, which stand out starkly from the surrounding grassy rolling hills, a very alien and massive industrial site. The byproduct of the mining, called slag, is piled in enormous ominous black mounds covering over 500 acres.[161] It is laden with cadmium, selenium, and radioactive radium, all of which can cause serious health problems including cancer in humans. It's unsafe to eat elk from nearby contaminated grasslands or fish from nearby waterways, including the selenium-polluted Blackfoot River.[162] The area is now an active Superfund site, meaning you, via your taxes, are helping to pay for the cleanup of the company's pollution, a business that earned over $2 *billion* in profits in 2018.[163] The phosphorus that is a component of glyphosate is also increasingly becoming a concern as a source of nutrient pollution where it is heavily applied – on corn, soy, and cotton.[164] Into Lake Erie, the Mississippi, and thousands of other water bodies it creeps. Consuming animal products drives demand for corn and soy, driving more of this greatest use of glyphosate, which is only one small component in the web of meat production. However, just this one factor has many radiating negative effects, many that come back to affect us. No pesticide has come remotely close to such intensive and widespread use as glyphosate, and it will take years to fully understand the full ramifications on our life.

A close runner-up behind glyphosate for the amount of chemicals applied to feed crop fields in the U.S. is another herbicide, atrazine. Based on reviewing hundreds of toxicity and ecological studies, the U.S. Environmental Protection Agency concluded that the chemical is affecting aquatic plant communities, and that there are risk concerns for birds, fish, mammals, reptiles, and amphibians where it is applied.[165] More than 400,000 pounds of atrazine wash out the mouth of the Mississippi River from farm runoff each year.[144] This is just two among many dozens of agrochemicals that are applied extensively to crops to supply livestock with food, and they all have effects on our ecosystem and us as the blood of life, water, connects us all.

All the corn, soy, and other feed crops that the United States, Brazil, and other countries produce on huge swaths of our best and often vulnerable soils both contaminate and consume vast amounts of freshwater, a resource becoming increasingly rare and contested. The production of meat requires enormous amounts of water, especially for the production of animal feed. Globally, agriculture accounts for 92% of the global freshwater we use, with 29% consumed or polluted to produce meat. Almost all of the water used to make meat goes into growing animal feed.[166] Beef and milk from cows leads the demand, using half of all the livestock water footprint. The water footprint for a piece of meat on a plate will vary strongly depending on where it was produced, what the animal was fed, and the origin of the feed ingredients. However, it uses far more water than plant-based foods. For example, the water footprint of a 150 gram soy-based vegetarian burger produced in the Netherlands is about 160 liters, but the water footprint of an average 150 gram beef burger is nearly 15 times larger, about the same amount of water an American would use taking daily showers for more than a month.[167]

The high level of water required to grow feed crops is contributing to the loss of critical groundwater supplies. Lying underneath the great plains of the United States is a massive underground lake, the Ogallala Aquifer. It covers portions of eight states and it supplies 30% of all the irrigated water in the nation. Water levels throughout most of the aquifer have dropped due to extracting water for irrigation faster than it is replenished by rainwater seeping into the ground. If it were completely drained, it would take 6,000 years to refill.[168] In places like Kansas, where the Ogallala Aquifer has been the major source of irrigation water, levels have dropped by 150 feet, forcing many farmers to abandon their wells.[169] Covering 50% of irrigated lands, corn is the number one irrigated crop in Kansas, and corn-fed cattle revenues far overshadow those from other agricultural sectors irrigated by its portion of the Ogallala

Aquifer. Other leading irrigated crops are wheat, grain sorghum, alfalfa, and soybeans, the latter three of these being primarily used for animal feed. Feed crop farmers in Kansas and many other regions are essentially "mining" a finite resource of water and converting it mostly to animal products. About 30% of the aquifer in Kansas was mined by 2010, and if extraction trends continue, eventually the amount pumped out can only equal annual replenishment. The existing storage of water, which took thousands of years of rains to fill, will be used up. Restricted to using only natural replenishment, farmers would only be able to pump out about 15% of the rate they extract now, a dramatic reduction in water use forced by its overuse.[170]

Another example of the extremely wasteful use of water for livestock is the production of alfalfa in sunny California, which helps feed the state's more than 5 million cows, primarily raised for dairy production. California alfalfa is also exported to Asian countries for the same reason. Over 90% of the alfalfa hay imported into China has come from the United States, with California being a key source.[171] A single gallon of milk from alfalfa-fed cows can require over 600 gallons of water to produce,[172] which is about the amount of water that would be used if you took a shower for nearly 5 hours straight. A 600 to 1 conversion ratio from one liquid to another is profoundly inefficient. In that great golden state on the left coast, alfalfa uses more water than any other agricultural use.[173] The state's number one agricultural commodity is milk, and it harbors one in every five of our nation's dairy cows. Growing hay and other forage and irrigating pasture for livestock accounts for 20% of the entire state's groundwater use.[174] Water for irrigation is commonly pumped from groundwater aquifers, but rates of groundwater extraction are unsustainable in many parts of the state. During drought years, which are likely to increase in intensity and frequency with climate change, up to 80% of the water used for irrigation in some alfalfa-growing regions comes from groundwater. The depletion of groundwater has driven the water out of reach of shallower wells that provide thousands of people with drinking water.

What a strange twist on nature and life to mine thousands of gallons of water, the most important resource of all, to be used on massive acreage of prime agricultural land to make one gallon of a substance that is at the center of causing widespread disease and death. And we are mining this precious water to foster the increasing consumption of dairy in China – even though most Asians are lactose intolerant!

~ Intensive Animal Production ~

Instead of grazing cows on open pasture as the "Happy cows come from California" ad campaign promoted, cows are now most commonly fed corn, soy, and other grain mixes in CAFOs. This method increases productivity and therefore decreases cost per unit of production. Although milk cartons may entice with pastoral scenes of joyful cows grazing on verdant hills, the reality of where most milk or beef is produced is drastically different. When you drive north on Interstate 5 out of Los Angeles and enter the San Joaquin Valley, you will soon come across a massive beef CAFO, the Harris Ranch. Able to hold up to 250,000 cattle, it is the largest in the state. You will smell it long before you see it. The acrid odor seeps into your car, a smell that is just repulsive. The concentration and processing of animals creates a massive amount of animal waste, which is why the stench lingers for miles downwind. Accompanying the stench in the air downwind of CAFOs are floating particulates of dried feces and urine, ammonia, and high levels of antibiotics and antibiotic-resistant genes.[175] The waste from the animals and slaughterhouse, like on many CAFO operations, is eventually diverted to storage lagoons and spread on adjacent disposal fields as a nutrient source. However, the loading of the waste on Harris Ranch fields, like many CAFOs, exceeds what crops can uptake. Excess amounts wash away. This has been a main cause for the underlying groundwater of Harris Ranch to have been found to contain nitrate in concentrations more than six times the federal drinking water standard.[176]

There are currently an estimated 1.6 billion animals in the 25,000 factory farms in the United States, producing an estimated 885 billion pounds of manure each year.[177] Our livestock produce seven times the amount of poop flushed down toilets by the nation's entire population of humans. However, unlike human waste, livestock waste receives little or no treatment before it is released into the environment. Like Harris Ranch, many of these operations produce far more waste than can be sustainably applied as fertilizer to crops onsite or nearby, creating excess runoff that pollutes soil and water. Nationwide, pollution from animal feeding operations threatens or impairs more than 14,000 miles of rivers and streams and 90,000 acres of lakes and ponds.[177] Like the nutrient runoff from corn and soy fields, waste runoff from CAFOs leads to excessive nutrients, algal blooms, and dead zones in downstream waterways.

North Carolina, which is the epicenter for hog production in the United States, is notorious for having massive lagoons filled with hog shit spill their banks during rainstorms, causing waves of pollution that spread and sicken downstream waters. The state's CAFOs are concentrated in the Coastal Plain, vulnerable to large storms. About 20% of them are located within 100 meters of a stream.[178] Passing hurricanes threaten hundreds of lagoons. North Carolina has 9.7 million pigs that produce enough manure annually to fill more than 15,000 Olympic-sized swimming pools. Most of that waste is pumped from the lagoons and sprayed onto fields in amounts that commonly far exceed the ability of plants to absorb the waste.[179] The negative health effects of this spraying and the resulting air and water pollution predominantly affects communities of color as these unappealing and dangerous industrial sites are situated on cheaper land among poorer communities that have less political influence. North Carolina is also commonly stricken with harmful algal blooms driven by this animal waste pollution.[180] Cyanobacteria found in blooms can make people and pets very sick. State officials warn that "toxins produced by cyanobacteria can affect the kidneys, gastrointestinal tract, liver, and nervous system of people, pets, livestock and other animals." The state's

Department of Health and Human Services offers guidance on how to keep kids and pets safe from toxic algae blooms, with a long list of warnings:[181]

- *Keep children and pets away from waters that appear discolored or scummy.*
- *Do not handle or touch large accumulations ("scums" or mats) of algae.*
- *Do not water ski or jet ski over algal mats.*
- *Do not use scummy water for cleaning or irrigation.*
- *If you accidentally come into contact with an algal bloom, wash thoroughly.*
- *If your pet appears to stumble, stagger, or collapse after being in a pond, lake or river, seek veterinary care immediately.*
- *If your child appears ill after being in waters containing a bloom, seek medical care immediately.*
- *If you are unsure whether or not a bloom is present, it is best to stay out of the water.*

I suggest one more be added to the list:

- *Eat less pork and other animal products.*

However, pork production generates massive income and therefore tax revenue for North Carolina, so it is unlikely the top health agency would ever recommend addressing the ultimate cause of this water pollution or human health crisis as it helps pay for their salaries and elects the government administrations that oversee them. It is a travesty that something that should be as carefree and fun as swimming or fishing in your community river on a hot, sunny day could be so hazardous to your and your family's health that "it is best to stay out of the water." That is the tradeoff for cheap pork consumed in copious amounts. If the water doesn't sicken you from the outside, cardiovascular disease is patiently working away from the inside.

The concentration of animals in CAFOs requires high levels of antibiotic applications to combat disease, but most antibiotics are added to feed to promote faster growth. This excess use fosters antibiotic resistance in pathogens that affect not only the livestock, but humans as well. CAFOs, due to their crowded conditions, are petri dishes for the future emergence of new infectious diseases and antibiotic-resistant forms of existing diseases. Constant monitoring of CAFOs, the livestock and handlers of CAFOs, and live animal markets is critical as these are the most likely epicenters of future pandemics.[182] These antibiotics and resistant microbes become part of the wastewater streams from CAFOs that enter the environment. Natural and synthetic steroid hormones found in CAFO waste can also reach groundwater aquifers and surface waters through a multitude of pathways. These hormones as pollution can have drastic effects on fish and other organisms, as well as contributing to breast and prostate cancer in people.[183]

The concentrated manure, antibiotics, and hormones that are continuously dispersed from CAFO locations across the world, and their potential for disease emergence, can be easily remedied. So can the over-extraction of wildlife, fish, and groundwater, as well as soil loss, forest loss, and ecosystem degradation that radiate out from our food choices. Ultimate causes reveal the ultimate solution.

Chapter 8: **Riding the Woody Wagon**

Vegan. What do you imagine when you picture one? Someone self-righteous. Smug. Elite. Un-American. Weak. It's a word many people instinctually recoil from. Vegans must be a little weird, right? Fitting the stereotype, the first vegan I ever knew was from California. He surfed. He hugged trees. He wore hemp. He smoked weed. The first time we crossed paths, I was, I admit, a bit disgusted. It didn't happen at a café in Hollywood sipping tea or in a yoga studio in Santa Monica. It happened one morning in the 1990s while sitting on a toilet in Costa Rica. I was busy doing my business, watching a lizard stalk a butterfly perched on one of the airy split-bamboo slats that formed the walls of the stall, when someone quickly hustled into the stall next to me. I have experienced diarrhea many times traveling in developing countries, usually from drinking water tainted with microbes. After a cringe of wishing I was not there to bear witness to the moment, I felt a sorry camaraderie for the soul splashing away next to me. He seemed quite unfazed, passing the moment with upbeat humming, and even letting out a whispered "damn" when he finished and must have witnessed the damage he did to that bowl. I had to bite my lip not to laugh. As quickly as he started, he was done, bolting out for a day of fun and surfing in the tropical sun. Anyone would be excited to start a day in this paradise, even after that. Life truly smiled upon that vegan.

Those bamboo toilet stalls, always scampering with wildlife, stood within an oasis of gardens down a shady dirt road, perched on the edge of the Pacific Ocean, and nestled near the tip of the Osa Peninsula of Costa Rica. This was my first visit to Tierra de Milagros, Land of Miracles. It was developed by three friends, Brad, Nikki, and Kia who transformed a former degraded cattle pasture into a bountiful retreat from the world. It was a place for their family and friends with problems − mental illness, drug addiction, or disease − to come rest and heal among the power and beauty of nature. Kia, a beautiful long-blonde-haired woman with strong features weathered from a life overcoming challenges, was the spiritual heart of Tierra. I often came across her topless, tan, and smiling as she tended the garden at the center of Tierra. Years later, she left to start an orphanage near Machu Picchu in Peru, after discovering children there sleeping in doorways and living in alleys strewn with human feces. Casa de Milagros, today known as Niños del Sol (ninosdelsol.org) is another testament to Kia's desire and dedication to heal the Earth and its people.

Next to the garden at Tierra was the Casa Grande, a towering conical structure with a thatched palm roof, its perimeter held aloft by raw wood posts. No walls connected those posts, but instead hammocks swung between them, creating a circle that was relaxed, open, and connected. The interior peak of the roof was held up by a central giant erect timber, its base enveloped by a large round wooden table for communal dining. Melted candle wax encased much of that center pole and the heart of the table in drippings. Connected to the Casa Grande was an open-air kitchen with long wooden counters made from thick single raw-cut pieces of wood, worn with use. It was the only place with an electric light, fueled by a single solar panel. The rest of the property consisted of a half-dozen small open-walled thatch-roofed huts reached by wandering down sandy paths through green shady tunnels of blooming pink and red hibiscus. Each hut was outfitted with a simple rustic bed under white mosquito netting and a table with a puddle of candle wax frozen in time. Just outside each hut was a shower, loose gravel for the floor, and a showerhead made from a coconut shell with holes drilled in it. Privacy was provided only by the surrounding lush vegetation. Water came by gravity from a nearby stream. A path through a canopy of guava trees led down to a beach, surrounded by black volcanic rock, that looked out over a perfect turquoise surf break.

It takes a bit to unwind, relax, and blend into the pace of Tierra, which over the ensuing days I finally felt. But that first day, I was still nervous and unsure about life and a decision I was on the verge of making. I had traveled to Costa Rica again, this time with an invitation from my friend, Jon, who was a volunteer along with me a couple years earlier in the Amigos program. After that summer volunteering had ended, Jon returned to live in Costa Rica and started up a very successful expedition company on the Osa Peninsula where he took visitors from the U.S. on hikes in the jungle and kayak trips through its waterways. I used to collect his newly purchased kayaks in my apartment in Miami before he stuffed them full of gear for the flight to San Jose. Jon lived in a very rustic former gold miner's shack that he bought, and visiting with him was always a journey to remember. His hair was long and his feet were bare, and he was an incredible host and cook for anyone that journeyed with him. These were the very early days of ecotourism, and his friendly, giving nature with a genuine smile enabled Jon to blaze a pioneering, adventurous path. He had settled in a small town on the outskirts of the country where arguments among inebriated men at the local bar sometimes descended into machete fights.   I once brought Brett for a visit during spring break of his final year at the Air Force Academy. Brett had rented a 4x4, and after spending a week travelling around the country, we stayed with Jon for a few days of adventure. On one evening, the local police officer, nicknamed "Rambo," pulled us over on a dark, dirt road. Rambo was so drunk he could barely stand up as he stared into the open window aiming an M-16 at Brett. He slurred words so sloppily in Spanish that I could not follow, but Jon calmly and gently coaxed the barrel of the gun down. Savvy negotiation and slipping Rambo a $20 bill was all it took for Jon to effortlessly handle the role of ambassador and solve another problem, one that could have ended very badly.

By word of mouth, Jon developed a list of clientele from the entertainment and business worlds who were looking for unpretentious connections with nature. National news anchors, Hollywood executives, and top actors were exposed to the magic of Costa Rica by Kayak Jon. My first trip to Tierra was to meet with one of them. I was considering leaving my doctoral program, after three years of studies and the seagrass research I was doing in the Florida Keys, to move to California. Jon had asked me to come and launch a rainforest conservation charity that a client and now friend of his was interested in creating. That friend was Woody Harrelson.

When I finally met face-to-face with Woody, I realized he was the same guy happily plopped next to me on the toilet that morning. It was a bit intimidating meeting him, even after sharing a moment of the most equalizing of bodily functions. He was a top celebrity who at the time was best known for his role as Woody Boyd on the massively popular TV show *Cheers* and leads in box office hits including *White Men Can't Jump*, *Natural Born Killers*, and *The People vs. Larry Flynt*, the latter role for which he received an Oscar nomination. He was paid many millions of dollars for starring in movies and had the capacity to spend that money on all the trappings that fame and fortune could buy – sports cars, mansions, planes – all the bling. But here he was, living off the grid, shirtless and barefoot in Costa Rica, and sitting down with a long-haired expedition guide and a young ecologist to talk about putting his money toward saving rainforest. We only had a few minutes of his time each day to talk business, as he was there to be away from all the attention that celebrity brings. About a dozen other people, including his wife Laura, were at Tierra to slow down, reflect, and live the pura vida. Decisions came slow with lots of reflection.

During mornings we were greeted with a symphony of birds and serenaded by the deep booming calls of howler monkeys.

Smoking weed, hiking the hilly jungle trails, surfing, yoga, and swimming in the ocean were the main tasks of the day, highlighted by some of the most amazing meals I had ever eaten – made only from plants. Upon carved wooden serving planks lined with the deep green of banana leaves were piles of fruits, veggies, salad, beans, and rice in a rainbow of colors, much of it harvested from the garden and trees around Tierra. Bananas, mangoes, papaya, avocado, pineapple, and passionfruit fresh from the earth were magnificent. They quenched the tropical heat. Rice and plantains were the carbohydrate fuel and beans nourished with protein. Coconut, garlic, onions, and ginger flavored and stewed many meals. At night, we ate under the glow of dozens of candles spiraling and dripping down the center post of the Casa Grande. Later a bonfire in the center of the circular garden drew us in for evenings of drumming or listening to someone strumming a guitar, all looked down upon by an explosion of stars against a pitch-black night sky. Bedtime was a cold shower to momentarily pause the sweat, naked in nature, and then reflecting on life by candlelight under mosquito netting. My mind still buzzed with weed and wonder from truly glorious days in paradise. I am deeply grateful for being invited into that private world, and to Woody for the paths his passion and support opened in my life. By the time I left for home from my first visit to Tierra, Woody told us he would donate a million dollars for us to start a charity to protect rainforest and pull together advisors to help steer it. As much as I learned from the experiences of developing that organization, Oasis Preserve International, in the end nothing impacted me as much as the lessons and examples I learned from Woody regarding food, even if I did not recognize it at the time. Wisdom also comes slow with lots of reflection.

Over the next couple years, we raised more funds by hosting dinners in Los Angeles and Miami where Courtney Love, Ziggy Marley, and Darius Rucker entertained. Depositing checks handed over from people, including many actors like Jennifer Aniston and Brad Pitt, was rewarding and a bit daunting, as we were entrusted to make an impact with their money. These were friends and colleagues of Woody who gave because he asked, and I know that also put a burden on Woody. It's never easy asking for money. A board of directors made up of leaders in entertainment, finance, and science joined the team, and they mentored our efforts. As a small organization we focused on supporting conservation projects in just Peru and Costa Rica where the team had experience and where conservation was vitally important. In Peru, we helped start the development of the Amazon Conservation Association, led by leading tropical conservation biologist Dr. Adrian Forsyth. The seed money that Woody provided helped establish one of the most successful conservation reserves in the Amazon, the Los Amigos Conservation Reserve, including the most active biological research station in the Amazon, fashioned from an abandoned gold mining camp. The trips I made to help scout the property with Jon, Laura, and my then wife and Oasis partner, Eileen, were thrilling and difficult. We once were on the verge of being lost at sundown deep in the forest, our guide nervously uncertain of the route back to our tents. If we went the wrong direction, we could walk for weeks, maybe months without seeing modern civilization – if we survived. On another trip, the relentless heat and humidity, constant sweating, and tremendous amounts of rain prevented my clothes or body from ever drying out. After a couple days, I developed a fungus on my skin, concentrated in my groin from the chafing of hiking, that made my skin flare, break, and bleed. I slept solo in my dank tent, legs spread eagle after a painful dousing of rubbing alcohol, but leaving the jungle for the drying respite of an electric fan in a town several hours away by boat was the only thing that halted the infection. The rainforest is exploding with life seeking nourishment, and I fed the mushrooms that time.

Being mentored by Adrian was a great honor, and revealed to us the most effective ways to raise and spend the very limited dollars that our society allocates to preserving nature. Few people on the planet have been as effective at conservation efforts. He had spearheaded the Amigos project following a career as a biologist studying under the famous E.O. Wilson at

Harvard University and later as a scientist at the Smithsonian Institution. He has published nine acclaimed natural history books and has developed four other biological field stations in the Amazon and in Central America. Adrian was the guru of the board with the experience and strategy, and he was very targeted with efforts to raise funds. Money is the fuel required to drive conservation projects. For several years he had been cultivating Gordon Moore, the founder of Intel, to support efforts to preserve large swaths of the Amazon. Adrian wanted protected areas that would contiguously link forests from the high Andes down into the flat basin. At the time, most computers were powered by Gordon's processing chips, which made him extremely wealthy – a whale of a potential donor. The money Woody donated helped get the Amigos ball rolling, and Adrian had told us to keep a look out for another check in the mail. It was an incredibly inspiring day when we opened a small hand-written envelope, with a folded personal check inside, written in cursive. It was for $350,000, signed by Gordon Moore.

A few years after we received that check, Gordon started a foundation with over $5 billion of Intel stock, half of his wealth. He has since donated just shy of $500 million to Amazon conservation efforts, helping conserve over 170 million hectares in the Amazon – an area more than four times the size of California.[184] The foundation has given billions in total to global efforts to protect ecosystems. For many years later, Adrian helped develop Gordon's foundation and has been integral to many global conservation efforts. Large portions of the Amazon have been protected due to the efforts of the Amazon Conservation Association (ACA) to establish conservation areas, address threats, safeguard indigenous areas, strengthen land management, connect habitats, and build climate resilience. ACA estimates "the current deforestation level of the Amazon at 17%, and its tipping point at 20-25%. If the tipping point is surpassed, the largest rainforest on Earth could become, at best, a dry grassland."[185] The forest is quickly approaching its tipping point. Even with the tremendous amounts of money donated by a caring billionaire, far more attention from more people and more funding is required. The simplest way to support the effort is by making a few changes in your diet. To get more directly involved, you can learn about the profoundly important work they are doing and/or make a donation at amazonconservation.org.

On the Osa Peninsula of Costa Rica, which was the wild-west last frontier of the country, the projects we supported successfully halted illegal logging by funding guards to patrol forests, setting up checkpoints for illegal logs leaving the peninsula, and lobbying the government to improve and enforce environmental laws. The people who worked the front lines risked the most, as they faced death threats for impinging on someone's income source, illegal or not. We had also laid the groundwork for collaborating with a cooperative of dairy farmers to try and improve the way they produced milk, incorporating permaculture practices into their lands. This would involve reforesting portions of their farms while incorporating rotational grazing on a smaller area subsidized with nutritious tree cuttings. All these pastures were created in recent years by clearing the forest, mostly in the hills, and the effects were tremendous on erosion, groundwater loss, and downstream reefs. Rust-red gully erosion scars were rampant in their fields. On the multi-generation farm of the leader of the cooperative, a freshwater spring that had bubbled crystal-clear water and flowed to the ocean had completely dried up. The oasis where he swam among tropical fish and crayfish during his childhood was now just a dry grassy depression in a hot field of wandering cows. Without the forest in the hills above, the water stopped percolating into the ground, which was the source of that spring.

Even in a place that can receive *20 feet* of rain in a year, without the sponge-like forest around, springs can run dry.[186] On several hours-long snorkeling trips to survey the coast of the gulf below, I could not find a single living coral. Large areas of dead reef were buried inches deep in soft mud. The deforestation and cattle grazing had taken their toll. As a proponent of permaculture (featured in Chapter 10), I was excited about this project. However, Woody, as a firm vegan did not want to support the production of animal products at the time. I was upset with the final decision to forgo investing in the project, but with hindsight I have respect for Woody's decision to stick with his principles. He did not want to personally finance animal products, especially those carved out of rainforest. The limited money we had was better spent keeping primary forests standing, and my ensuing years have revealed clearly that eating less dairy and meat is the key to addressing expanding pastures and fostering their reforestation.

Perhaps the most profound lessons I learned riding the Woody Wagon, as we called his entourage of characters, were those that related to food. Before I moved to LA, I ate as I had for most of my life before. Vegetarian options were not very enticing where I came from. They meant a plate of bland veggies, either raw with a ranch dip or steamed to mush with not much else. I was never exposed to vegan cuisine made with expertise, intention, and dedication. As I soon learned, it can be both incredible and terrible. Those first experiences at Tierra had exposed me to the explosion of amazing flavors and great feeling that consuming copious amounts of freshly harvested fruits and vegetables can create. The sun, surf, and weed heightened the experience no doubt. As we spent time hanging at Woody's houses up in the hills above Hollywood or down near the beach, new ways of looking at food and nutrition arose. I had never tasted spirulina before, a blue-green algae loaded with protein and nutrients. Straight up, it was not palatable, tasting like grassy fish, but mixed with maple syrup, tahini, almond butter, lemon juice, and cinnamon into a bright green dripping paste and poured over a bowl of cut fruit topped with coconut flakes and chopped nuts, it was incredible. "Painted fruit" is a favorite of mine to this day and always leaves a green smile. Mixed into a smoothie, spirulina adds a deeper flavor, protein, nutrients, and a purple color. Massive, delicious salads made from a diverse mix of greens and sprouts as the center of a meal became imprinted in my palate and still are a staple on a nearly daily basis. I learned delicacies can be made with tofu, tempeh, cashew-cream sauces, and that avocado could add smooth richness to just about anything. Woody's kitchen revealed the magic of fresh-squeezed juices made from a rainbow of fruits, veggies, and wheatgrass sprouting from trays like green carpet on the countertop, all churned out from a humming white Champion Juicer. The same machine could churn out frozen "ice cream" made only from frozen bananas and other fruits.

The experiences I had around vegan food, however, were certainly not always delicious nor ones I wanted to pass on to others. At the time, eating only "raw food" was a diet fad just beginning to sprout in California. Raw food is not cooked, never exceeding a maximum temperature that varies among different interpretations of the diet, but generally not above 118° F (48° C). No baked breads. No crispy crusts. No cooked pasta. No cooked veggies. No steaming bowls of soup. No golden-warm chocolate-melting cookies! Raw food diets may include raw fruits, vegetables, nuts, seeds, meat, eggs, honey, and unpasteurized dairy products. A small group of people, without scientific support, claimed that raw food was more nutritious and invigorating because it still contained all the natural enzymes that were broken down in the cooking process and it was best to only eat raw food. They wrote books about it. A movement arose around the concept. Restaurants opened, including one financially backed by Woody and Laura. O_2, as it was called, was located on the Sunset Strip, in the heart of the Hollywood nightlife. It served non-alcoholic herbal drinks, raw food, and offered oxygen on tap that you could inhale like an emphysema patient through silicone tubing that mounted into your nostrils. The increased oxygen levels were supposed to benefit my health as well. No doubt it was much healthier than breathing Los Angeles air, but I never felt any effects from the O_2. I remember years later wishing I had it while I was mountain climbing with Brett. Some of the drinks were really delicious and unique, but most people out on the Strip were looking for alcohol. A couple of items on the raw food menu tasted pretty good, but many were just too extreme. Raw food tends to be very dense and heavy with flavor, and without cooking it often has a mealy, grainy, or pasty consistency. And when all food is never raised to high temperature, it's boring. You just can't make a satisfying "crust" from uncooked nuts.

On many nights after visiting O₂ during its opening weeks, Eileen and I would make a stop on our way home to grab a sizzling mushroom pizza, well-done and golden with real cheese and a crispy crust. I was still walking the line of veganism, and delving into the extremes of raw pizza made with a dense, mealy room-temperature crust just made me run the other way. O₂ did not stay open for long, as most other people seemed to have a similar reaction. Raw food can be tasty, and is beneficial as part of a diet, but not an exclusive diet. Studies have since revealed that a strict raw food diet could lead to being underweight and that nearly one-third of the females under 45 that were studied experienced partial or complete loss of their menstrual cycle due to nutrient deficiencies, and therefore a strict raw food diet should not be recommended for extended periods of time.[187] Many foods benefit from cooking – not just for flavor and texture but also to release vitamins and minerals. A central problem with the raw food theory is that the human body already supplies the enzymes needed to digest and absorb foods, and the enzymes in food are largely inactivated by the acidity of the stomach.[188] A healthy and tasty balance between cooked and raw is what makes food taste best…and better for you. Of all the vegan places I have dined, my favorite, and also a regular stop for Woody, was *Real Food Daily*. They nailed it with home-style and healthy, especially their mashed potatoes and gravy. I wish they were everywhere.

Business pioneers often get the arrows. It takes brave people to open frontiers. A healthier restaurant is not easy, especially surrounded by a sea of alcohol and animal products. As donors, entrepreneurs, and influencers, Woody and Laura have been amazing pioneers and leaders in supporting and promoting environmental and health solutions – hemp, veganism, legal marijuana, protecting old growth forests, and helping others to share their voices. Woody took real risks. He hung off the Golden Gate Bridge on a rope to draw attention to logging of our last great old-growth forests in the northwest U.S. –

something I would not try in my wildest dreams. When hemp was still illegal, he planted their seeds in Kentucky, getting arrested for a gesture that helped spearhead a hemp and marijuana industry now widely legal, worth billions, and promoted by U.S. Senators. Woody was challenging to corral into meetings most of the time, as he genuinely was enjoying a very free-flowing and fun life of a celebrity, and many of those meetings started with sparking a joint. The life of a successful actor can be a great life and no wonder thousands of people head to Hollywood seeking it. However, he was equally serious and dedicated, and very intelligent. He was driven and had worked hard, sleeping on friends' couches for years while auditioning for endless acting roles for which he was turned down. Never giving up, he achieved wild success in pursuing his dream career, and it was inspiring to see up-close someone with such large financial and social capacity giving their attention to positive solutions that may seem out on the fringes at the time, but turn out to be very important. He could afford large cash donations to our planet, stylish hemp outfits, and someone to prepare amazing vegan food. Decades later, many of the solutions, products, and businesses he supported are now becoming mainstream and far more affordable. Shifting diets to protect the environment is now critical, something he foresaw decades ago.

Near the end of our ride on the wagon, Eileen and I had Woody, Laura, and their toddler daughter Deni over for dinner in our home. We lived in a tiny apartment in Venice Beach. The kitchen counter was 2 feet wide. As we crafted plants into a feast, Woody played hide-and-seek with Deni. Even in the tiny shoebox of our home, Woody was humble, creative and playful. In light of all I have learned since about food and health, I look back on that evening of laughter, thankful for crossing paths with a wise and powerful vegan who embraced and valued life. Many forests remain standing and countless species still exist because of him, and his knowledge and passion has radiated out through many people to the benefit of all life. He has promoted the business of natural, which for most of society is unnatural.

The destruction of nature around the world is largely fostered by the power of business, the draw of wealth generation by for-profit enterprises. The goal is to maximize profits, and by reducing costs, one can help make a business even more profitable. Food production has become built around this model, with costs reduced by pushing them onto others. For example, a farmer who cuts a forest and plants corn to feed livestock has a goal of maximizing yields and producing the crop as cheaply as possible. Laying down fertilizers and spraying pesticides helps achieve this, and the farmer pays money for those ingredients in his production model. However, a portion of the fertilizer is not taken up by crops and the excess and much of the pesticides are washed away into waterways, a disposal of waste that is not paid for by the farmer. It's a "free" disposal, and the ultimate costs are borne by society in the form of algal blooms, toxic waters, fish kills, and negative financial effects on fishing, tourism, and drinking water. The CO_2 the farmer released into the atmosphere when he cut and burned the forest is another free disposal route with societal costs of climate change and sea level rise, and the myriad of expenses that are associated with them. There is no charge for the biodiversity erased with the forest, even though it may contain information of great value to humans – maybe something far more valuable than Taq polymerase. The loss of habitat for birds, insects, mammals, or fish that contributes to the beauty and magic of life for everyone is not paid for by the farmer. You may value seeing monarch butterflies fluttering past your giggling children, but the widespread use of pesticides exerts a cost on you by making those experiences far rarer. It costs you and your children in quality of life, not the farmer nor any of the customers down the line, including you, in cash now. The fossil fuels burned in the production of the agrochemicals, farm equipment operation, and groundwater pumps also release CO_2 into the great free dumping ground of the atmosphere. The farmer is not charged money for the groundwater mined, but the price is paid by others when wells run dry. Here in the U.S. we further reduce costs for corn and soy farmers through federal subsidies for their insurance and also ensuring that farmers are paid at least a minimum price for their products in case market prices fluctuate low – all paid for with your tax dollars.

Reducing costs for corn and soy growers via externalized waste streams and tax subsidies is the underlying reason you can buy a fast-food burger or rib sandwich for just 99 cents. We all pay more for that burger indirectly through rivers with toxic algae that can kill your pets, water you can't drink or swim in, or when you pay Uncle Sam your taxes every year to help keep the polluting, water-hogging industry afloat. At the heart of modern agriculture is a very linear model fueled by oil and natural gas. Fossil fuel is extracted, burned, and adapted into agrochemicals to grow crops, all of which spew waste in a myriad of forms out of the production system – a cost borne by all of us. This is the opposite of the tight, cyclic, solar-driven systems of nature.

During one of those nights nibbling on raw food at O₂, the way I looked at conservation suddenly and energetically changed. It came with a very bitter and green taste in the mouth. It was as if a lightbulb dimmer turned up high in my mind, fueled by caffeine and vitamins, that illuminated the power of markets to drive conservation. Two brothers introduced themselves to me with a big hug. David and Steven Karr, smiling and kind, came with a book of photos telling a story. But before opening the book, David opened a bag of what looked like ground-up ganja. He scooped what were crushed leaves and small stems into a hollowed-out polished tan gourd. Its outer surface was zigzagged with intricate dark carvings. He then inserted a silver metal straw into the gourd, the *bombilla*, the bottom of which was flattened like a spoon and covered in small holes. From a thermos, he poured hot water into the greens and held out the gourd to me for a sip. From the end of the straw, an explosion of grassy and smokey bitterness rolled down my throat. The first sip was not pleasant. It was strong and bitter. I choked down a few more sips until the straw chortled with air. He took the gourd back, refilled it with water, and passed it on to the next person. Around a small circle it went. By the time it returned to me, the bitter shock had calmed and become slightly pleasant. I also noticed that my mind had become more active, I was smiling, and the conversation flowed easily. Around the gourd went, again and again over the next hour of chatting, and every so often David would pack it again with fresh leaves for a burst of fresh bitter energy. It was my first experience drinking yerba maté and I was honored that it was from a place of such reverence for not just the beverage, but for its ultimate roots – the rainforest.

Steven flipped open the photo album and told us the story behind the drink and their company, Guayakí Sustainable Rainforest Products, which they had founded together with three other friends, including the Paraguayan visionary behind the company, Alex Pryor, who came up with the idea as part of a college senior project. Yerba maté, commonly referred to as just maté, is made from the leaves and small stems of the yerba maté plant, *Ilex paraguariensis*. It is the national drink of Argentina, Paraguay, and Uruguay where it is consumed for its energizing caffeine boost instead of coffee. It is consumed hot or cold as *tereré* from gourds, carved wooden cups, or hollow cattle horns. Every gas station in the region has a hot water dispenser for people to fill their thermoses. Most of the crop consumed in those countries is grown, like coffee, on giant monoculture plantations under the sun. Forests were felled, linear fossil fuel production systems set up to maximize yields, and many costs – deforestation, soil loss, chemical use – externalized to the public and planet.

However, Guayakí Yerba Maté was grown in the shade of a rainforest reserve in Paraguay, in the sub-canopy habitat where the maté plant is found in the wild. It was harvested by native Guayakí people, providing excellent jobs and good working conditions. The smokey hue of Guayakí Yerba Maté comes from a unique recipe of tropical hardwoods extracted and burned from the reserve, the smoke passed through the leaves during the drying process. New hardwoods were replanted to take their place. Selling their maté would generate income, creating value in the standing trees, and help protect and fund the future of the forest reserve. The model was pioneering, and in the coming years the product would become a hit in the U.S., growing steadily from its groovy west coast roots. In the early years, they served up samples at natural food stores and music festivals from a hand-painted VW bus, often with still-dripping surfboards inside.

Eileen and I eventually joined the Guayakí team and helped develop the company in its early years. Approaching the Guayakí Rainforest Reserve was like coming upon a mirage-like island in an open and empty sea of tilled soil. Over 95% of the forests of Paraguay have been razed to the ground, lands now filled to the horizon with pasture and soy for livestock. Entering the forest reserve was journeying into a magical and precious ark, a shady labyrinth where jaguars roamed and birds still sang in abundance. It felt like journeying into a secret world in a movie – dappled, unfamiliar, and drawing the eyes to find hidden beings that were probably watching us. In a small portion of the reserve, scattered among the towering trees, were maté plants. Birds jumped among their branches, and insects crawled and buzzed about. That island of forest not only produced tremendous wildlife and acted as a giant oasis soaking up and making rain, but it also grew money on trees from its healthy soils.

Americans loved drinking Guayakí for the feeling it gave, immediately from the caffeine, vitamin, and mineral kick, but also because customers want to support something good. The wave that started on the left coast spread across the country. With continued market demand and reinvestment, the company launched bulk packaged teas, tea bags, bottled and canned beverages, and energy drinks, tamed and flavored to better appeal to the American market than the gourd and bombilla. As demand for maté increased, it drove the planting of more production trees, and this offered an opportunity. Maté trees could be established in deforested areas, planted along with many other species to create new forest with maté grown in the shade below to fuel its protection and further expansion. Using the power of the market, the company was slowly, methodically helping bring back the Atlantic Forest. An extremely endangered ecosystem, it is characterized by very high biodiversity and endemism, with 40% of its vascular plants and about 60% of its vertebrates found nowhere else in the world. The Atlantic Forest used to run in a continuous strip along 2,000 miles of the eastern coast of South America from Brazil to Argentina but has been reduced to only 15% of its original extent and only 7% if you include just the viable fragments at least 100 hectares in size.[189] The forest is home to around 20,000 species of plants. Some 450 tree species have been found in an area that would cover just over two football fields[190] – a staggering amount considering the entire United States contains only about 650 tree species.

Today, Guayakí has a central mission of Market Driven Regeneration™ which at its core involves developing long-term partnerships with indigenous peoples and small farmers to harvest yerba maté from the rainforest and forested farmland at fair trade prices. This helps fund the farmers' economic sovereignty and land stewardship, preventing further deforestation of critical forests under threat from political and economic forces. Upon this foundation are other company principles including generating zero waste, net zero greenhouse gas emissions, and social justice. Guayakí Sustainable Rainforest Products offers a simple market-driven approach: the more you enjoy and purchase their products, the more positive impact you make. From a small start-up among a group of surfer-friends, the company now has tens of millions of dollars in revenue, stewards 174,000 acres of forest that protects over 400 species of plants and animals, providing $140 million in ecosystem services.[191] With "board meetings" floating on surfboards off Central California, camping among a Guarani tribe, and serving up maté at parties in Hollywood mansions, it was enlightening and inspiring to have witnessed the pioneering and fun spirit of a for-profit business model that proved to be incredibly successful and valuable for both people and planet. Doing well by doing good. It is a great example for others to emulate. Many food, beverage, and other companies could apply similar strategies. Profits driving good. The nourishment we put in our mouths, sell, or offer to others can have dramatic impacts, positive or negative. The choice is up to us.

More than a decade after we enjoyed that incredible and eye-opening ice cream made from frozen bananas in Woody's kitchen, Eileen and I were on the verge of trying to bring that same treat to the rest of the world – and feed ourselves in the process. During the four years leading up to the 2008 global financial crash, we had dedicated our time and money to developing a start-up healthy-lifestyle company, Nui. We had launched a beverage into national distribution, published the first in a planned series of youth eco-adventure books, and were in negotiations to develop a cartoon series with the goal of inspiring kids to solve health and environmental problems. A series of food and media projects geared to youth were in the works. Business was looking up. We were going to do well by doing good. In the middle of a multi-million-dollar capital raise, we had traveled to Aspen, Colorado to meet with a billionaire that was interested in our company who we thought would be the final member in the fundraising round. However, while we were having lunch at our hotel the day before our pitch, the TV news announced that stocks had precipitously dropped. The assistant to the investor called to say our meeting was pushed back a day. Then two. Then three. Then it was cancelled. He had lost tens if not hundreds of millions of dollars during those few days of market decline. Every investor pulled out of our deal. Money sources of every type were frozen. It took us four years to build that business, but just four months later, we closed. We soon lost our home, our life savings, and had to borrow money from family to survive. The kindness of a friend put a roof over our heads. With one piece of luggage each, Eileen and I lived in her guest room for a year. We did a lot of cooking to pass the time.

During those months of reflection, I had scratched out an idea for a kitchen appliance based on that magical fruit ice cream maker from Woody's kitchen. My version did not make juice, but only those frozen treats. I believed if I could make a machine that served up healthy ice cream, one which cost $50 instead of $350, we might be able to sell some and get back on our feet financially. After many meetings, calls, and beers, we convinced a childhood friend of mine, one who had built a successful business manufacturing products and selling them into major retailers, that it would be worth the risk funding this idea and taking it under the umbrella of his company. About a year after the global financial meltdown, we had one fragile protype of the device, manufactured on a 3-D printer and spray-painted to look like it came off an assembly line. We had called in favors to produce an infomercial, which we wrote, directed, and shot that would air as a test on cable TV channels. Before investing the massive expense of producing inventory, our business partner was going to risk significant dollars buying ad space on TV to test the waters – to see if people would call in and order from what we called a "faux-mercial" – as we had only that one single delicate machine. However, as Eileen and I eagerly anticipated the day that those commercials were scheduled to air, doubt came knocking.

The broker with whom we had been arranging the purchase of air time for our commercials had called with concern and a touch of pity. She said, "You two seem like really nice people. I want to help you out. We haven't seen a kitchen appliance have success in years with an infomercial. This product is never going to sell. You are going to lose your money. I recommend cancelling this. Find something else to pursue."

We hung up the phone devastated. Eileen cried. We had pinned our hopes on this to get us back on our feet, under our own roof again. We thought about it, but not for long. Our guts told us we were onto something. We never told our partner about that call. We ordered the air time, and nervously awaited the day the first ad would air. Astoundingly, the orders flooded in. Within a year, we were selling millions of Yonanas® all over the world, trying to spread the decadent pleasure and health of plant-based diets. It became a top gift pick of Oprah and Dr. Oz. Over several years, Eileen traveled to dozens of countries, from Malaysia to Brazil, to introduce it into local cultures. Hundreds of flavors and recipes were created – from my American holiday favorite, pumpkin pie, to flavors created in Japan with seaweed. The messages we received from customers were humbling and inspiring, especially those who shared how the product changed their health. People suffering from lactose intolerance, obesity, diabetes, and even cancer wrote touching notes to us giving thanks for our creation and passion for sharing this ice cream made only from plants. That entire business and all the people around the world who enjoyed and benefited from Yonanas was inspired by hanging out in a vegan kitchen – tasting, learning, and sharing.

Our palates, when pleasured, are powerful forces that can ripple around the planet. And jumping on a wagon into foods unknown can take you on amazing journeys.

Chapter 9: **Predicting the Future**

Change can come fast. Very fast. Just 30 years ago, when *Cheers* was the number-one TV show in the United States, I used to swim in a crystal-clear Biscayne Bay next to the Miami skyline. It was a beautiful undersea world filled with undulating, bubbling seagrass beds and schools of bonefish, spotted eagle rays, and horseshoe crabs. It had looked like that for many thousands of years. Today much of the bay is a brown, murky wasteland with a fraction of the wildlife remaining and frothy decay collecting on its edges. During this very month of August, 2020, people are trying to ward off an ongoing fish kill and extensive toxic algal blooms by pumping air into the bay using fossil fuel-powered generators like a giant aquarium aerator.[192] The seagrass used to pump out that oxygen, and suck up carbon dioxide in return. Increasingly higher water temperatures hold less oxygen and also turn up the metabolism of animals, which drives the need for more oxygen. It becomes a death spiral. Like a ventilator on a Covid-19 patient with a raging fever, we are trying to inject life-giving oxygen into a bay on the verge of flatlining. Nature used to do it for free and reward us with a bounty of beauty and fish. Change to our collective human health can happen just as quickly. Only 30 years ago, about one in 10 people in the U.S. were obese.[193] Today it's four in 10.[28]

What will life look like in 30 more years? Will more of our waterways and coastlines be inundated with rotting and toxic algae, starving of oxygen, closed to swimming, boating, and useless for fishing? Will most of the coral reefs have died off or degraded into stark barren remnants of their former bounty, their fisheries that support billions of people collapsed? Will we still have a giant, expansive Amazon forest or will it be a sea of soy, grass, and cows? Will a never-ending list of species that have been crafted into their uniqueness by millions upon millions of years of thriving and evolving be snuffed from our planet forever? Will the rest of the world catch up to America's staggering obesity, diabetes, and cardiovascular disease levels? Making predictions is fraught with uncertainties, but historical trends, recent data patterns, and simple mathematics can help estimate where current trends may lead us. We can estimate effects and anticipate potential consequences. Perhaps enough of us will recognize the outcome as unappealing and we will change our habits and alter our path toward a better life. If we don't, life on Earth will soon be dramatically different and the damage will be nearly impossible to reverse.

As much as climate change makes headlines, I believe it is critically important to focus on the loss of biodiversity. Many threats facing our environment and us may seem enormous and devastating, but in fact they are relatively simple to address and reverse. For example, the underlying cause of the damage in Biscayne Bay is primarily local nutrient pollution. Excess phosphorus and nitrogen are leaking from human waste in septic systems and fertilizers running off lawns and agriculture, directed into the bay by canals. Even mansions that cost tens of millions of dollars put their poop in septic systems that continuously leak nutrients into the environment. Rapid runoff from hard surfaces – roofs, roads, parking lots – which have expanded in the last few decades, also funnel polluted water into the bay via those same canals. Bringing water clarity back to the bay requires stopping those sources. It is an easy fix. Septic systems should be quickly phased out. Fertilizers and pesticides should be banned from lawns. Hard surfaces should require water runoff storage and infiltration technologies, all of which can readily be installed. If the water quality returns, so will the grass, oxygen, and wildlife. It may cost a few billion dollars to achieve, a decade to roll out, but the damage can very likely be quickly reversed. Even climate change can be halted and likely reversed if we switch to sources of energy that are not fossil fuels. This must be driven by political will and R&D support by governments for solutions that act against ingrained, powerful industries that currently make massive profits off coal and oil. The livestock sector contributes about 15% of global greenhouse gas emissions, equivalent to all emissions from transportation, and shifting our diets will help address climate change as well.[194] However, with biodiversity loss, the damage cannot be undone, even by spending trillions or working at it for hundreds of years.

When biodiversity – genes, species, and the ecosystems they comprise – is eliminated, we cannot bring it back. We will never even know that many species or the valuable information they contained even existed before they are gone. The exuberance of life forms and ecological interactions that make up our planet today have been shaped by nature for eons through the craftmanship of nature, a force of beauty and magnificence that we cannot remotely come close to replicating. We will hang human-painted artwork, which we value at hundreds of millions of dollars, in museum vaults guarded by alarms and arms to preserve the original image. However, only a well-trained eye could tell a replica Mona Lisa from the original. If the original was burned, it would have zero effect on our lives. None. A replica could easily take its place for humans to gaze upon. The Yangtze paddlefish species is truly one of a kind and there is no replica. It will never be seen again. We cannot make replicas of animals, ecosystems, or the interactions of their trillions of genes once they are gone. We are allowing them to be pilfered from our planet. Stolen from the next generations. How greedy we are. We already feel their absence, and their further disappearance will reverberate around the world. Our climate, water, food, and medicine – the stability and abundance of life – are rooted in the biodiversity of life. Our life.

When biodiversity disappears, it is gone forever. Most of our biodiversity occurs in the tropics – the developing countries of the Americas, Africa, and Asia – far from the lives of the wealthier nations of North America and Europe. The future of biodiversity in the tropics looks very precarious. The continued grandeur of nature is quickly deteriorating in countries where populations are booming and their diets are rapidly changing to emulate richer developed nations. Much of the content of this chapter is adapted from my Ph.D. dissertation, *The Role of Agriculture and Food Consumption in Tropical Conservation* as well as the article, *Conservation: The Key is Reducing Human Carnivory,* published along with co-authors Dr. Kenneth Feely and Dr. William Ripple in the journal *Science of the Total Environment.* Highlights of the research were also published in *Science, Nature,* and the *Proceedings of the National Academy of Sciences,*[195] which are considered the three top scientific journals in the world. Achieving that trifecta reflects the importance of this subject within the minds of science, a force which strives to understand the world in order to better guide our future.

The historical pattern of what has driven habitat loss is very clear. Over the 300 years ending in 1990, the extent of global cropland area increased more than five-fold and pasture areas increased more than six-fold. Pasture for livestock now encompasses an area on Earth that is 3.5 times larger than the entire United States.[196] Although some agricultural expansion is driven by farmers growing crops for direct human consumption, livestock production, including feed, uses approximately three-quarters of all agricultural land and nearly one-third of the ice-free land surface of the planet. *It is by far the single largest use of land by mankind.*[99] Though difficult to quantify, animal product consumption by humans is likely the leading cause of modern species extinctions, since it is not only the major driver of habitat loss but also a principal driver of land degradation, pollution, climate change, overfishing, sedimentation of coastal areas, facilitation of invasions by alien species, and the loss of wild carnivores and herbivores.[197]

Feeding the largest river by volume in the world – 11 times the output of the Mississippi – is the Amazon rainforest. It is the planet's largest tropical forest and is a profound example of biodiversity loss being driven by livestock production. Though it covers only 4% of the Earth's surface, the Amazon contains a third of all known terrestrial plant, animal, and insect species. Never before has so much old-growth and primary forest been converted to human land uses so quickly as in the Amazon region. This rapid change has been driven overwhelmingly by demand for livestock. Over three-quarters of all deforested lands in the region have been converted to livestock pasture and feed crop production for domestic and international markets.[198] Rising worldwide demands for meat, feed crops, and biofuel are driving rapid agro-industrial expansion into remote Amazon forest regions. A recent brief period occurred in the late 2000s when deforestation rates slowed in the Amazon as soy production expanded more into pasture and was offset by the similarly devastative clearing of native vegetation in the adjacent Cerrado region. However, rates have again increased in the Amazon. Eventually, cleared land that is suitable for feed crop production will become scarce and any remaining forests outside of protected areas in the Brazilian Amazon will be at risk of conversion to soy. An upsurge of deforestation for livestock is now occurring even in protected areas.[199]

In some other biodiverse tropical regions, the livestock industry is not a leading factor in deforestation. For example, in Africa, timber harvesting and fire appear to be the two main processes leading to deforestation, with instances of farms replacing forest predominantly due to small-scale cropping.[99] However, a rise in feed crop production is projected for Africa as international agricultural companies are acquiring or leasing land in Africa to grow them for export markets, modeled after the industrial development of the Brazilian Cerrado region.[200] Hunting of wildlife as a bushmeat source is considered to be a more immediate and significant threat to the conservation of biological diversity in many African and southeastern Asian tropical forests than deforestation, which as discussed in Chapter

5 also causes many cascading trophic effects.[201] Hunting, habitat modification, and denial of access to water and other resources by humans, in combination with competition and disease transfer from livestock, are driving critical declines in wild herbivores.[52]

Agricultural production in tropical Asia, which has transformed natural habitats for thousands of years, is based primarily around the intensive production of rice and wheat and other secondary crops. Multi-purpose livestock are integrated with many crops in small-scale farming systems that characterize historical agriculture systems in Asia. This integration intensifies total food output, and the closed, recycling nature of these mixed farming systems makes them less damaging to the environment. However, in many Asian countries, all of the available arable land is nearly completely utilized. Under growing demand for meat by urbanizing populations, livestock production is rapidly changing in Asia, with both an increase of production and a shift away from mixed farming systems to CAFOs located near urban markets. This drives negative environmental consequences of increased monoculture feedstock demands at local and international scales as well as increased pollution of surface water, ground water, and soils by nutrients, organic matter, and heavy metals.[202]

Because of its devastating effects on natural habitats and species, land-use change is projected to continue having the largest global impact on biodiversity, especially in tropical forests where societies are increasing animal product and feed crop production.[203] The health of many of the world's poorest people living in developing countries would be improved if they could include more essential fatty acids, minerals, vitamins, and protein in their diets. Combating malnutrition could be achieved by both animal- and plant-based sources.[204] However, livestock has been the primary focus for increasing protein supplies. The rapid expansion of livestock production in developing countries has been referred to as the "livestock revolution."[205] As incomes in many of these countries, like Costa Rica, have grown in recent decades, per capita consumption levels of animal products have also increased, including high growth throughout the tropics.[206] Half of global meat production now takes place in developing countries, where the amount of meat each person eats per year on average more than doubled from 24 lbs. (11 kg) to 55 lbs. (25 kg) from the early '70s to the late '90s.[99] With continued economic growth, meat consumption by citizens in some developing countries can be expected to quickly approach levels found in high-income industrialized countries of between 176 lbs. (80 kg) and 286 lbs. (130 kg) per year.[207]

Animal products currently comprise about one-fifth of the weight of all food eaten by people on Earth, which is a 24% increase since the 1960s. However, great disparity exists among developed and developing countries. Animal products make up almost half of the food consumed in many richer nations. The United States, many European nations, Australia, and Argentina are prime examples. This is contrasted with the majority of sub-Saharan countries and most of Southeast Asia, which have had a consistent pattern of low animal product consumption, making up around 10% of their food. Of concern are the historically low, but rapidly increasing, rates found in several countries throughout Asia, Africa, and South America – most notably China, which has quadrupled the amount of animal products from 5% to 20% of their diets since the 1960s.[208] People eating more meat combined with rapidly growing populations in most developing countries will be the potent force driving much more habitat and biodiversity loss.[209] Much of the projected future population growth will occur in the most biodiverse tropical nations. Today the tropics contain about 40% of the global human population, but house over half of all children under 5. By 2050, it is expected that more than half the world's population will be in the tropics, containing over two-thirds of its young children, and adding 3 billion people to our current global population of 7 billion.[206] All those new hungry mouths will require protein, and the source of that protein will have profound effects on everyone.

As part of my dissertation research, I estimated the effects that increasing meat consumption will have in countries that contain most of the world's biodiversity. Across global ecosystems, 25 biodiversity hotspots have been identified that collectively contain, as endemics, approximately 44% of the world's plants and 35% of terrestrial vertebrates.[210] These species are found nowhere else on Earth. These hotspots formerly covered only about 12% of the land surface of the planet. Due to destruction by people, the total extent of these hotspots has been reduced by nearly 90% of their original size – meaning that this wealth of biodiversity is now crammed into less than 2% of Earth's land surface. Among the top five hotspots for endemic diversity, the Caribbean has lost 90% of its primary forests. Its downstream coral reefs have also been heavily impacted by this conversion and most are a whisper of their former glory. Madagascar has lost 90%, the reason its soils bleed into the ocean as if its skin had been cut off. Brazil's Atlantic Forest has lost more than 90%, which puts in perspective the importance of the pioneering work of Guayakí. The combined southeastern Asian regions of the Malay Peninsula, the islands of Borneo, Java, and Sumatra and their surrounding islands, have also lost over 90%, much of the deforestation also driven by production of palm oil, a key ingredient in processed junk food sold worldwide.

Just 17 countries together harbor over half of the Earth's total species, a small fraction of our global collective of 193 nations.[211] Fifteen of these megadiverse countries are developing countries located in the tropics, and two are rich and developed – the United States and Australia. The historical dietary patterns of these 17 countries reveal great inequities and trends that could have profound consequences. Below is a map of megadiverse countries that indicates the change in their Human Trophic Level (HTL)[208] over about half a century from 1961 until 2009. In an ecosystem, a trophic level of 1 are the primary producers (plants) that fix sunlight into biomass. Level 2 are the herbivores that eat only plants. Level 3 are the carnivores that eat the herbivores. Levels 4 and 5 include apex predators that eat herbivores and other carnivores. Consumers at each trophic level convert on average only about 10% of the chemical energy in their food to their own tissue (the 10% energy law discussed in

Chapter 5), and therefore ecosystems rarely have more than a level 5. All the energy fixed by the primary producers, with 90% lost at each step up the food chain, is used up after five levels. Nothing is higher up the chain than a great white shark, because there is not enough energy left to support an even higher predator. Like bears and chimpanzees, human beings are omnivores. We eat plants and herbivores, and consume only limited amounts of other carnivores (for example, fish that consume other fish). When calculating in every type of food we eat, the HTL lies between a level 2 (herbivore) and 3 (carnivore). As a species within our global ecosystem, our HTL is 2.21, indicated by the dashed line. This number, which means that roughly 21% of our food comes from animals and 79% from plants, varies dramatically among nations. What stands out are the two bookends, the U.S. and Australia, which get about 45% of their food from animals. This is a drop from 50% a half century earlier, a slight trend in a good direction, but still too high and dramatically higher than many other nations. A consistent trend of increasing HTL is seen across most megadiverse countries over time. Increases in the two most populous countries in the world, China and India, are very concerning.

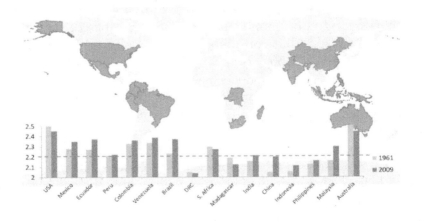

In order to attempt to gaze into the future and see what effects changing diets in developing megadiverse countries might have on biodiversity, I examined the amount of land needed to make different types of meat, how much agricultural land a country currently has, and projected changes in the amount of meat each country is projected to consume years in the future. The results estimate how much new land will be required to meet the total meat anticipated to be produced in 2050 for each country. To me, the results are astounding.

Developing tropical megadiverse countries would need to expand their agricultural land base by an estimated 3 million km^2 by 2050 to meet projected increases in meat production. This is an area of increase equivalent to about one-third of the entire size of the United States to supply new meat production in just 15 countries. It is a massive area that would be developed for making livestock. To meet these meat production expansion needs, developing countries will need to clear out more nature. They are also acquiring land in other countries as well as selling or leasing land within their borders to fulfill other nations' food demands.[200] Because of changing dietary habits and increasing population, China will have enormous effects on biodiversity far beyond its own borders. From 2000-2030, China will likely add over 250 million new households, which is the equivalent of doubling the number of households in the entire Western Hemisphere that existed in 2000.[212] Currently about 20% of China's food consumption is animal product-based, near the global average,[208] but consumption of animal products is on a trajectory to reach 30% only 20 years later.[82] Already over the past 20 years, animal products have increased from 10% to 20% of Chinese diets, and were only 5% in 1960. By the turn of the millennium, each person in China on average consumed four times more meat and milk and eight times more eggs than they had consumed just 30 years prior.[212] If China eats like Americans, which is possible in the next 30 years or so, each of its projected 1.5 billion inhabitants would more than double the amount of meat and other animal products they currently eat.[212]

Despite rising animal product demand, the extent of agricultural land in China has been decreasing under pressures of urbanization and land appropriation for mining, forestry, and aquaculture. As in the United States, grasslands in China have been severely degraded by overgrazing and other pressures, with 90% of the nation's grasslands now considered degraded. Production rates of grasslands have decreased approximately 40% since the 1950s.[212] Consequently, China's increasing appetite for animal products will need to reach far beyond its own borders to meet its needs, importing both meat products as well as feedstocks to produce meats locally in CAFOs.[202] Much of the livestock production in China is fueled by soy produced in the Amazon, with annual imports of soy from Brazil growing from zero in 1996 to 60 million tons in 2012.[82] Approximately 4.2 million hectares of Brazilian cropland is utilized for exports of soybean to China for livestock feed, an area about the size of Japan.[213]

Projected increasing demand for animal products in developing megadiverse countries, like China, could potentially be met by increasing supplies from other regions with lower biodiversity. However, the effects of animal product production beyond potential biodiversity loss (soil loss, biocide use, etc.) are important even in lower biodiversity areas. In addition, current trends, including the large supply of soy to China from the Brazilian Amazon, indicate an expansion of sourcing of agricultural products from tropical developing countries. Land grabbing, the transfer of the right to own or use land from local communities to foreign investors through large-scale land acquisitions, mainly for agriculture, has increased dramatically since 2005. The increase began initially in response to the 2007-2008 global increase in food prices and growing food demand (especially in China and India). In just two years from 2008-2010, the World Bank estimated that about 45 million hectares had been acquired by foreign investors, an area larger than California.[200] Grabbed areas are often in developing tropical countries with sufficient freshwater resources and often are a large fraction of a country's land. This loss of land to fuel meat consumption in other richer countries takes land away that could feed local mouths. Given current population and dietary trends, the extent of land area converted to agriculture to meet growing global food demand could drive a loss of 1 billion hectares of natural habitats in just the next few decades – *an area larger than the entire United States!*[214] This land will be carved out of the last tropical frontiers of the Americas, Africa, and Asia. The Amazon. The Congo. Indonesia. Malaysia. Papua New Guinea. The wild lands of Earth. Our biodiversity.

The globalization of the food trade, production of foreign feed sources, and standardization of food products is driving the replacement of wild and biodiversity-rich traditional agricultural lands with extensive monoculture landscapes. Crop diversity and knowledge about these plants found within traditional mix-cultured systems is threatened by this industrialization.[215] In addition, the biodiversity found within crops of traditional farming systems is decreasing as industrial agriculture expands, driven by a global system of uniform, unblemished foods that ship and store well.[216] In the early 1900s in the United States, commercial seed houses offered hundreds of varieties of each type of vegetable crop, but today the numbers have plummeted. For example, lettuces decreased from nearly 500 varieties to just a few dozen. The biodiversity of our crops, the unique genetic information carried in thousands of varieties, is key to developing strains that can be more resilient to disease or changes in climate. Also essential is the knowledge of local farmers who foster and evolve this biodiversity. As many people in wealthy, developed nations have come to appreciate locally grown, farm-to-table, and diverse artisanal foods, far more of the world is quickly moving in the opposite direction toward industrialized farming, animal-centric fast-food diets, and global food systems controlled by a small group of very large, very profitable companies that will export as much of their costs to you and your environment as possible.

Without changing our dietary trajectory, we are on a collision course for losing massive portions of ecosystems on our planet where the expression of life is at its greatest. Our lives, and those of our descendants, will be diminished by its loss. It is not just how people eat in the developing countries where biodiversity lies, but it is our collective food culture, often led by corporate powers of America that will determine its fate. We cannot expect the world to continue with a few rich countries gorging on and profiting from meat, and others increasingly trying to copy them. Our planet will experience a collective heart attack, wheezing and struggling against chronic inflammation to keep life pumping through its ecosystems. Ultimately, change is the decision of the individual. It is your decision. It is your life.

Chapter 10: **Solutions**

The enormous presence of livestock in our lives can perhaps be better grasped by looking at it in terms of how much everything weighs on the entire planet. Of all the mammals here on the third planet from the sun, we humans make up about 36% of the weight. Wild mammals – elephants, whales, lions, bears, bats, deer, rats, and all the other warm-blooded furry creatures that total about 6,400 species – make up just 4% of the weight. Our livestock, made up of a dozen or so species and dominated by cows, pigs, and chickens, comprise a staggering 60% of the weight.[217] As most of the energy in plants is lost as it passes through that livestock to us, even a small increase in the consumption of animal-based foods will drive a large increase in plants required to feed the livestock. With at least 3 billion more hungry mouths likely to come, and billions already alive and on a trajectory to eat more meat, this will drive widespread habitat conversion, greenhouse gas emissions, soil loss, pollution, and irreversible biodiversity loss. That small percentage of wild animals will decrease even more as humans and livestock increase. Peeking into the future for just the developing megadiverse countries in the last chapter gave just a small indication of that loss. We could very easily continue on that trajectory. Your children may live in a drastically different world where spectacles of the Amazon, the Serengeti, the Congo, and Borneo — and their priceless life forms like pink river dolphins, lions, elephants, and orangutans — are only legends of the past. Those places will live only as electronic memories in documentaries and words in Wikipedia, experienced blandly and fleetingly through smartphones and TVs with the last lonely specimens found in zoos or behind chain-link fences. The vast majority of Americans, and likely many other cultures soon to follow, will be viewing these images, thumbs clicking away on bodies that would struggle to walk through those places if they even existed, held back from vitality by the excess fat that envelops their bodies and riddles their circulatory systems with disease. It looks very likely that this will be our outcome in less than one more human generation.

However, just as fast as negative change has come to shape our ecosystems and our own physiques, we have the capacity to alter our trajectory. The solutions are astoundingly simple. It will involve sharing and inspiring change, both at a very personal level with the ones you love, and among global cultures. At the core is celebrating life. Ours and that of our fellow species. As individuals, we will need to make choices. Personal choices, very simple to make and delicious to execute, are the key to a healthy, prosperous future for all. I propose we make three: Reduce. Replace. Reintegrate.

~ Reduce ~

If we want healthy thriving bodies and ecosystems long into our future, we have to eat less processed junk foods and drinks, less meat, less eggs, less dairy, and fewer fish. Period. However, we don't have to stop eating them. You can scratch the idea of having to go vegetarian or vegan from your mind. Though it is definitely the healthiest option for your well-being and the planet's health, it is not remotely realistic to sway you, millions of our fellow citizens, let alone billions of people, to eat *only* plants. However, reducing consumption is the foundation on which our future must be built. Reducing demand for livestock products, or other demand-side mitigation measures, such as reducing food waste, offer the best potential for meeting the challenges of feeding our burgeoning population while limiting biodiversity loss and greenhouse gas emissions. For the sake of argument, what would happen if everyone on Earth did decide to turn vegan to reduce health costs and stave off that long list of environmental problems? Eliminating the loss of energy available in plants that occurs through livestock production and instead growing crops only for direct human consumption is estimated to increase the number of food calories available for people from our current agricultural lands by as much as 70%. We could feed an additional 4 billion people, exceeding the projected 2 to 3 billion people to be added through future population growth, all from existing farms and fields.[218] No more cutting rainforest. No plowing under more grasslands. The Amazon, the Congo, and many other biodiverse lands could remain untouched, wild, evolving.

Substituting soy for meat as a source of protein for humans would reduce total biomass from the planet converted to food by humans in 2050 by 94% below what was consumed in 2000, because by eliminating 90% of energy wasted going from plants to livestock, we would need less crops to feed us all.[219] Soy and other legumes are excellent sources of protein, can be turned into many types of food products, and meet complete amino acid dietary requirements.[220] Recall that when compared to an equivalent mass of common raw cuts of meats, soybeans are protein powerhouses. They contain on average twice the protein of beef, pork, or chicken, and 10 times more protein than whole milk. When comparing the area needed to produce 1 kg of protein from soybeans (12 m^2) to the average land area required to produce common cuts of meat, chicken requires three times more area (39 m^2), pork nine times more area (107 m^2), and beef 32 times more area (377 m^2).[221] Few choices our society makes will have as great an impact on our future collective health as reducing the amount of animal products we eat.

Equally important at the forefront of any reduction should be powerful efforts to lower the amount of food we waste. A staggering amount of food is wasted worldwide, especially in developed nations. In the United States, 30% of all food, worth more than $48 billion, is thrown away each year.[222] My young guide Carlos in Colombia would have appreciated the smallest bites of that. Reducing this waste, especially related to animal products, would impart profound environmental benefits. Waste varies greatly between countries, especially developing and developed. For example, daily food wasted in India for vegetables and pork is less than 3 calories per person, dramatically less than the daily waste of 290 calories per person for beef in the United States. Beef that is never eaten is not only calories wasted, but causes all those cascading negative environmental effects. All that damage for nothing in return. Because of the level of our waste and the level of animal products in our diet, about seven to eight times more land is required to support food waste in the United States than in India, even though India has almost four times as many citizens. The elimination of food waste in China, India, and the United States combined is estimated to be able to feed over 400 million people per year, which could feed more than everyone in the United States.[223]

Meat, dairy, and eggs can still be a part of human diets as reducing consumption and waste can still allow for some livestock production, especially on lands where it is appropriate. Traditional plant-based diets combine legumes and grains (for example, rice and soybeans in Asia and rice and black beans in Latin America) to achieve a complete and well-balanced source of amino acids for meeting human physiological requirements.[224] Although veganism is growing in popularity, completely eliminating animal-based products from global diets is not only too simplistic and impractical, but it does not make the best use of many land types.[215] It is estimated that grazing on pasture unsuitable for growing any crops, and which did not cause deforestation, contributes approximately 14% of total global livestock feed.[225] Some of that pasture should still be used to make livestock, albeit with wise rotational practices that regenerate soils, protect waterways, and sequester carbon as well as ensuring substantial areas of grassland are available for sustainable populations of wildlife. In small-scale farms, especially in poor cultures with marginal lands unsuitable for many agricultural crops, livestock are a valuable resource that converts low-protein grass and other plants into more concentrated protein in a self-transportable format and are also a vital form of insurance during hard times.[226] But reliance on livestock can be relieved by creating biodiverse local food systems and protein supplies based on plants.

Three basic facts face us regarding food and our future: (1) We need to increase calories and nutritional health for a growing, developing global population. (2) We need to dramatically decrease the land demands and ecological footprint of agriculture in order to maintain biodiversity and improve global ecosystem health. (3) Most people will still want to eat meat, dairy, and eggs.[227]

What is the best way to address this conundrum to maximize benefits – both health and enjoyment? By eating 90P: increasing plants in our diets to 90% of all the food we eat. *I propose that it is critical that we strive toward a goal of significantly reducing the amount of animal products in our diet, ideally to a global average of 10% or less of calories.*[195] *This could be roughly guided by limiting average daily consumption of animal products to include a maximum of 100 grams of meat (which is about the size of a deck of playing cards), three eggs, three slices of cheese, or two cups of milk.* Only one of these options in a day on average, or roughly combined on some days and balanced with other days eating only plants rich in protein, fiber, and nutrients. Chapter 11 lays out ideas on how to integrate this 10% limit in our diets. This upper cap on animal product consumption, combined with a reduction of food waste, would enable the future global population to be fed on existing agricultural lands, and we could potentially restore many habitats, especially forested lands that were converted to pasture or feed crops.[195] All this while people still get to enjoy meat at a much healthier intake level. Reaching these goals and reducing the overall global animal product consumption to about 10% of diets will require significant decreases in per capita meat and dairy consumption by developed countries and little or no increase in most developing countries.[208] *For developed countries like the United States, Australia, Argentina, and many in Europe, this will require us to consume only about one-quarter of the amount of animal products we now eat.* A deck-of-cards-sized 100-gram serving of cooked meat has about 25-30 grams of protein.[83] This is about half of the recommended intake of protein for an average man (56 grams) or woman (46 grams).[228] The other half of daily protein can easily be met from plant-based sources, which also contain fiber, a critically under-consumed dietary component that is also at the center of our healthcare crisis. People in the United States consume, on average, twice the daily recommended amount of protein.[229] With the amount of animal products developed countries now consume (40-45% of diets), far more protein is eaten than is needed for overall health, contributing excess calories to obesity and heart disease, and being flushed away by hundreds of millions of people as excess nitrogen-rich waste in toilets. Biscayne Bay, and many other polluted waterways, are the ultimate effect of that excess.

If enough people can become aware of and value the massive personal and environmental health benefits that shifting their dietary choices can create, perhaps we can succeed. I believe we should be hopeful. Great success has previously been accomplished in changing some dietary habits that are extremely damaging to wildlife. A notable example is the recent campaign against consumption of shark fin soup in China. The soup is made from the strands of cartilage that provide the underlying structure of a shark's fin. When boiled and shredded, they look like noodles and add texture and thickening to the soup. Offering negligible nutritional benefits and no flavor, the shark fin as the base of a soup is driven primarily by tradition. It is served as a luxury item and a common menu item at celebrations like weddings and banquets. With over 1.4 billion people in China, that equates to a lot of celebrating and enormous amounts of shark species consumed, many highly endangered. It is estimated that 100 million, potentially more than 250 million, sharks are killed annually, with parts from three-quarters of them ending up in shark fin soup.[230] It would take piling up the equivalent of 14 of the largest U.S. warships, Ford-class aircraft carriers, to equal the weight of sharks killed annually.[231] A huge proportion of these sharks are caught, their fins cut off while they are still alive, and then tossed back into the ocean to sink and slowly die. A cruel waste of both meat and life.

A large-scale media campaign featuring Chinese National Basketball Association star Yao Ming and other Chinese celebrities in social media, television, bus stop, and billboard advertisements was disseminated widely throughout China in 2006 and again in 2009. Messages focused on the declining numbers of sharks and their important role in the ecosystem, the cruelty involved in the practice of finning, and the presence of mercury in shark fin soup. Surveys found that 83% of people exposed to the campaigns had stopped or reduced consumption.[232] The Chinese government pledged to ban shark fin soup from official banquets. Conservation organization WildAid claims that there was a 50-70% reduction in shark fin consumption over a two-year period during the campaign.[233] Recent Chinese government statistics reveal an 80% reduction in consumption, as well as 81% declines in the country's shark fin imports in some of the largest cities between 2010 and 2014. Unfortunately, the success in mainland China has been offset by increasing shark fin soup consumption in other places like Hong Kong, Macau, and Thailand, and increased consumption of shark meat in countries like Brazil.[234]

Eating sharks, like livestock, is also bad for personal human health. As apex predators at the top of marine food chains, sharks accumulate the highest concentrations of toxic substances such as mercury, methylmercury, cadmium, and arsenic as they consume and concentrate these poisons from their prey, acquiring more the longer they live. This also occurs in other predators like marlin and tuna. Long-term exposure to these toxins can cause cancer, skin lesions, cardiovascular disease, and neurological impacts.[234] Predators and nearly all species of marine fish are also consuming copious amounts of plastic waste in the ocean, and the health effects are just beginning to be understood but will likely reveal many unforeseen negative outcomes.[235] As with shark fin soup in China, animal product consumption is ingrained into many societies. High levels of livestock consumption are a traditional part of many diets or a sign of affluence in many countries. One advertising campaign echoed this cultural tradition in the United States, "Beef: It's what's for dinner." Meat is often believed (incorrectly) to be a physiologically necessary or superior form of protein. Many cultures also consider livestock ownership to be a sign of higher status.[226] In addition, as in the United States, many governments financially incentivize livestock production and animal product consumption over plant-based foods.[99] The connection between livestock consumption and its subsequent ecological damage is less direct than with shark fin soup, but achieving a similar level of decline is not impossible.

Clearly many challenges exist, but awareness is increasing. According to a Gallup Poll in 2020, nearly one in four Americans said they ate less meat in the past year than they had previously, while three-quarters said they ate the same amount of meat. This decreased consumption is driven primarily by personal health concerns.[236] People want to live better. They want to thrive. Not just in the United States, but around the world. Even in Brazil, the largest exporter of beef in the world, the number of people who declare themselves vegan or vegetarian has nearly doubled over six years, comprising 14% of the population. During the past couple years, Brazilian plant-based food-startups have seen soaring demand.[237] Fueled by rapid urbanization, eating more animal products, and lifestyle choices, chronic diseases have emerged as a critical public health issue in China, as they have in many other developing countries. A decade ago, the Chinese government set a goal of promoting public health, making healthcare accessible and affordable for all Chinese citizens, and reducing chronic diseases by promoting healthy eating and active lifestyles.[238] In the end, success will be driven by one factor: personal choice. But choices are driven by awareness and understanding. Promoting traditional Chinese plant-based diets would benefit their people profoundly, and could set an example for other cultures to follow. The United States should do a much better job of promoting plant-based diets. It could be our easy, inexpensive evolution to better health and much lower healthcare costs. We will need political and cultural agreement around the globe. The two largest economies in the world, the United States and China, which are currently jostling for economic and political power in the depths of an animal-product-driven pandemic, could help everyone by agreeing on one thing: we should eat fewer animals.

~ *Replace* ~

Cows may rule much of the surface of our planet, but they provide us overall with a very small portion of our nutrition. Less than 5% of the protein consumed by people worldwide comes from beef and 10% from milk. This compares to about 6% from pork, 6% from seafood, 9% from poultry and eggs, and over 60% from plants – the real powerhouses of protein![239] However, the ecological footprint of beef is much higher than other meats. Land-use rates vary by country, but cows, which are a mixture of grazing and CAFO animals, require on average at least 20 times more area to produce a ton of meat than chickens and pigs. If cattle are raised only on feed crops, the area of land required decreases but is still twice the area required for pigs or chickens. Far more area is required on tropical pasture to produce an equivalent amount of meat, up to 100 times greater than feedstock-raised animals, which is why cutting rainforest to graze cows is so incredibly wasteful.[240]

Within the goal of reducing the proportion of animal products in our diets to 10% of calories, efforts to reduce beef and favor chicken or pork will magnify benefits to ecosystems and biodiversity. Beef should be an occasional treat, certainly not a daily or even weekly staple. We should be promoting "Beef: It's what's for dinner…very rarely." I eat it a couple times a year, and it is amazing when I do. In addition to the lower amount of land required to produce meat, pigs and chickens produce a fraction of the methane as cattle, sheep, or goats, which ruminate their food. Bacteria in their guts break down their food, releasing methane, which is burped out. Methane is the most abundant non-CO_2 greenhouse gas and because it has a much shorter atmospheric lifetime (about 12 years) than CO_2 (up to thousands of years), it holds the potential for more rapid reductions of climate change effects. Decreases in emissions could potentially be accomplished quickly and relatively inexpensively by eating chicken and pigs instead of beef and milk.[241] A shift of preference for meat products is already occurring and should be further supported. In developed countries, total livestock production increased by 22% between 1980 and 2004, but ruminant production declined by 7% while that of poultry and pigs increased by 42%. As a result, poultry and pigs make up over two-thirds of total meat production, and poultry is the meat with the highest growth rates across the world.

However, the best option for being able to foster lower meat consumption is by replacing it with something better. Something healthier, that requires far less resources, but most importantly – is delicious. We are incredibly intelligent beings that have achieved amazing marvels of biotechnology and engineering, and our inventive and entrepreneurial minds have just begun to tackle this problem. I have no doubt we are in for a rapid evolution of delicious and healthier foods that will take the place of meat, eggs, dairy, and even seafood throughout many channels of our food industry, from fast-food and school lunches to fine dining. Inventions and companies are being created and advertising dollars spent around innovative and delicious plant-based foods to replace many of our meats. Creative minds are rethinking how plants are prepared and served. Inventive chefs in pricier restaurants have even been crafting treats like watermelon "ham," the breakout star of plant-based charcuterie, which also has given rise to creations like radish prosciutto and jerky sticks made from burdock root.[242] Delicious plant-based food is poised for growth through many channels – with your demand. Demand drives profit. Profit will drive more options and better solutions. The free market is the answer.

In 2015, before the company became a multi-billion-dollar phenomenon, I had an opportunity to visit with Pat Brown, the CEO and founder of Impossible Foods. I met him at the company headquarters for a one-on-one discussion and reflection on markets driving positive human health and environmental wellness. Fitting for a former Stanford biochemistry professor in an office at the heart of Silicon Valley, Pat appeared casual in jeans, tennis shoes, and an unbuttoned red flannel shirt over a rainbow tie-dye Impossible Foods t-shirt. However, his mission was serious. He went on sabbatical from Stanford about five years prior, and during his year break he wanted to solve a big problem. As a vegetarian for more than 40 years and vegan for 10, livestock production was not only personal, but also one of the biggest environmental problems he thought could be solved with science. The problem was so enticing, he never went back to Stanford. He told me his goal was "to put the livestock industry out of business." After five years and a company valuation more than $5 billion, he is off to a good start with a half-percent slice into a livestock industry worth well over $1 trillion. Among the first to introduce burgers made from plants that taste and cook like meat, the company has been rapidly expanding its products in thousands of restaurants and grocery stores. An Impossible Whopper became a hit at the fast-food behemoth, and the delicious burgers can be found at many kinds of restaurants near just about everyone now.

Before he ever launched his idea, Pat first tested a theory. He believed even meat lovers might eat burgers made from plants if they tasted like real burgers. Making burgers as delicious and satisfying as the real deal would require lots of investment and brainpower. However, the scientific theory, and investors, needed an experiment that could offer some proof. His was simple. He sampled burgers to 600 mid-American meat eaters in 12 cities, 50 people per city. He gave them real beef burgers but told them it was made from plants. People thought they were delicious. When he surveyed the subjects, he found that if given the choice, 2.5 times more people would choose the burger they thought was from plants than a regular burger. When they were told the "plant" burger had no cholesterol, even more people chose the plant burger. He also discovered they would be willing to pay twice the price for the plant burger if it was delicious and pleasurable without the baggage of cholesterol and bad health. The lesson that came from those early experiments is that although there are some hardcore meat lovers that only want to eat animal meat, most people's desire to eat meat is not the desire to eat animals – they just want to eat delicious food. People are afraid that giving up meat is giving up pleasure. If you can successfully recreate the pleasure of meat from plants, *and* make it heathier, that could be a game changer.

If he created a better product, he believed he could outcompete the livestock industry. He felt the meat industry was vulnerable due to bad basic economics. Beef is low margin and its supply is unpredictable. Producers need to plan two to three years ahead of market need and have little agility to meet instability. As Pat explained to me, if you have a bad year as a beef producer, "you are fucked." His goal was to beat them on price and taste with plants. He can increase efficiencies and remove instabilities in production. He can also make meat taste better by eliminating non-pleasurable and bitter compounds like some amino acids that are found in meat. In the end, he can make it more delicious and less expensive. He started with burger meat because more than 50% of all beef in the U.S. is ground. Ground meat might seem pretty simple, but it is a complicated product to formulate. It is not completely uniform, but a blending of many types of tissue ground and mixed together. To replicate it, he had to make plant-based tissue-like products – connective tissues and fat cells – that when combined feel and taste like a burger. The product needed to replicate key sensory experiences that people value in ground beef. Its appearance, texture when raw, sounds and smells while cooking, and even the flowing bloody juices had to be part of the experience. He had to deliver on all expectations.

Pat approached three venture capital firms, pitched his idea, and raised start-up funds. Silicon Valley is a very special and unique place. It is close to capital, filled with talented scientists, but most important, it has a mindset like nowhere else that "you can invent a new world." Pat hired a team of 70 people to start R&D. A good scientist, of course, has knowledge in their specific field to tackle the biochemistry of the product, but what is harder to learn is solving problems. Being an entrepreneur pioneering new fields is all about learning how to solve problems. The team had to deduce the materials and compounds to replicate in meats, discover what plants would have the right proteins, and test plants to find the flavor molecules. All this had to be done affordably, competitively. The main flavor of meat comes from heme, which is found in hemoglobin, the protein in blood that carries oxygen. Heme contains iron molecules, which gives your own blood that slight metallic taste and its red color when exposed to oxygen. Plants also produce heme, found in the root nodules of legumes. At first, they extracted heme from legumes, but later developed a more reliable, less expensive, and more ecologically beneficial method of making it by engineering a yeast to produce it as a product. Yeasts make our beer, wine, sourdough, yogurt, and many cheeses. They have been engineered to make medicines and biofuels. Why not adapt one to make heme? By harnessing nature and utilizing the information in its biodiversity (and certainly using Taq polymerase during the process), the scientists of Impossible Foods solved the riddle. They are working on more. He had high confidence they can make anatomical structures like muscle tissue. Think steak. Bacon. Iconic American meats.

Since its founding in 2001, Impossible Foods has raised $1.5 billion in funding, and in addition to burgers and ground meat to replace beef, it has also developed products to do the same for pork. This could prove incredibly lucrative in China, and be key to reducing the ecological footprint of the country's rapidly changing diet. Today I went grocery shopping and stocked up on many of my favorite plant-based replacements for animal products that I had consumed for most of my life – burgers, chicken patties and nuggets, milk, cheese, mayonnaise. Pat now has many competitors – Beyond Meat and a recent favorite of mine, Dr. Praeger Burgers, being two successful examples. When we met five years ago, that is exactly what Pat said he had hoped for most of all – competition. He welcomed competitors working against the profoundly destructive livestock industry. "People doubted the automobile as a technology to replace horse and carriage. They thought there is no way horse and carriage could be replaced. They both get you somewhere. However, one does it with better efficiencies and pleasure." It may have started with Ford Motors, but competitors blossomed and evolved. Today we even have newbie Tesla, and the space continues to evolve for the benefit of mankind.

"The global devastation from the expansion of the meat industry is not coming," Pat told me confidently at the time. Like a chess game, he even planned ahead with his investors. The company had a central clause that it could never be sold to a meat or dairy company. Even though a sale could generate a huge payout and give Pat billions of dollars in cash, the product and patents could be shelved to drive more real-meat sales. I am confident his company and others like it will grow tremendously. The key isn't selling meat eaters meat. It's selling them plant products that are delicious. As I departed, Pat left me with a final nugget of wisdom. "We must make meat eaters happy. Our future best friends are hardcore meat eaters!"

Providing economical alternative protein sources to developing countries, such as some low-footprint animal products or innovative plant-based solutions, as soon as possible is key to averting extinctions of tropical wildlife.[201] In addition to curtailing the destructive livestock industry, we need to relieve pressures on hunting of wildlife as a protein source. We need businesses that emulate Impossible Foods or its competitors, launched within regional countries that could make plant-based products that best replace local wild protein sources. Consistent, reliable sources of delicious and inexpensive protein, with flavors to match local tastes, are an important part of relieving pressure on fisheries and wildlife while increasing food security. However, unsustainable consumption of wildlife also remains a problem even in many relatively prosperous countries with sufficient protein supplies as eating bushmeat in many places is considered a delicacy or a sign of affluence.[243] This is similar to the historical and cultural perceptions around shark fin soup in China which, as discussed previously, has been addressed with considerable success through public awareness campaigns. With innovation, investment, and marketing, societies can shift their values and diets. Entrepreneurs can make lots of money around the world with plant-based protein products. Better health and a better environment will be an investment return that benefits everyone.

As beneficial as many of these meat replacement products are, they still need to be balanced within one's diet. Many, including the Impossible Burger, are still high in fat (14 grams), including saturated fat (8 grams). That is one of the core reasons any real burger tastes so good. Our tastebuds love fat. However, an equal-sized burger made from standard ground beef that blends 70% lean meat and 30% fat contains twice as much fat (32 grams), and 50% more saturated fat (13 grams).[83] Just on fat content alone, plant-based burgers are far superior. Regarding environmental effects, the difference is astounding. Impossible Burgers use 96% less land, 87% less water, and produce 89% lower greenhouse gas emissions than real beef burgers.[244] Unlike beef, the Impossible Burger also contains no cholesterol, which is at the root of cardiovascular disease. A major bonus is that it also contains fiber (3 grams), which is an important benefit compared to beef, or any other meat, which harbor none. However, our diets need way more fiber than 3 grams. Total dietary fiber consumed from food should add up to at least 25-30 grams per day.[228] Eating 10 Impossible Burgers is not the way to achieve this as your body would be overwhelmed with 80 grams of saturated fat, four times the maximum daily recommendation. Most adult Americans consume only about 15 grams per day of dietary fiber. Obese individuals tend to consume less fiber than healthy weight people.[245] On a grading scale, this 50% achievement in fiber is a solid failing "F" for our nation. When it comes to our health, both physical and mental, fiber is perhaps one of the most important things we can consume. Achieving an A grade in that would revolutionize our health as it will foster vitality of our internal life forms –

organisms that equally match our own body's cells in number and importance.

At most you are only half human, composed of about 30-40 trillion cells containing your own DNA that make up your bones, muscles, skin, blood, nerves, and organs. Your alter ego is composed of about the same number of bacteria cells, maybe even more. Your very own microbiome. The number you harbor will depend on what you eat, your body size, age, ethnicity, culture, and the environment within which you live.[246] However, without these bacteria you would quickly die. Found all over the surface of your body – in the eyes, nose, mouth, under toenails – the 500-1,000 different species form different communities occupying the many ecosystems of your body. The vast majority, about 95%, are found in your digestive system, and they are key to your survival. If we gathered together all these bacteria from your body, they would fill about half of a soda can. In your gut, especially in the large intestine, they work in tandem with the enzymes our own bodies produce, breaking down food into its nutritional components to be absorbed into our blood and spread around to every one of our cells. They build and maintain us. They work hard and die fast. Whenever you look down at a coiling pile of poop in your toilet, about half of that brown mass is made up of bacteria that helped feed and protect you.[247] However, their ability to help you depends heavily on what you feed them. Fiber is paramount.

Intestinal bacteria facilitate their beneficial effects through the fermentation of dietary fiber to produce short-chain fatty acids, which have many important roles. A critical one is reducing inflammation. Inflammation is a natural process that helps your body heal from injuries and defend itself from infection, as when your ankle swells after a sprain or you experience a fever to fight off infection. However, when you have underlying chronic inflammation – for weeks, months, or even years – it can be very detrimental to your health. Dietary culprits that are believed to feed this inflammation and diseases associated with it are sugar and high fructose corn syrup, refined carbohydrates like white bread, vegetable oils and trans fats used in processed foods, and red and processed meats.[248] Fiber-rich foods, which fuel a healthy microbiome, help suppress the incidence of and mortality from many inflammation-linked Westernized diseases, notably cancers of the colon, breast, and liver; cardiovascular, infectious, and respiratory diseases; diabetes, and obesity. Reduced fiber and its effect on the microbiome is believed to be closely associated with the swelling population of patients with obesity and type 2 diabetes in the United States, Africa, and China. A healthy gut microbiome is also believed to be tied to mental health, including cognitive health, ADHD, Alzheimer's disease, depression, anxiety, and stress.[249] Microbiomes present in vegan intestinal systems have been shown to harbor low amounts of bacteria normally present in meat-eaters that are responsible for converting L-carnitine, a compound in red meat, into a chemical – trimethylamine-N-oxide (TMAO) – that greatly increases atherosclerosis.[250] Omnivorous people that eat red meat daily are shown to produce significantly more TMAO than vegans or vegetarians, a process dependent on gut bacteria. Being primarily vegan, and eating meat only occasionally, your body may not harbor enough of the bacteria that can create TMAO. Our gut microbiome is critical to our health, and lots of research is ongoing about the positive effects of fiber and plant-based diets.[251] Certainly, many exciting discoveries await. In the meantime, one truth is clear: as societies shift and eat more animal products and processed foods, they eat far less fiber. This happens because animal-based protein sources lack fiber, whereas plant sources, especially when eaten as whole foods, are just packed with it.

Throughout your life, you may have been told to eat fruits and veggies as an important source of fiber, but far better are the protein-rich plant products – legumes and whole grains.[83] Following is a list of plant foods and their percentage of fiber by weight raw:

Legumes		Grains		Roots		Vegetables		Fruits	
Soybean	9%	Maize	7%	Potatoes	2%	Asparagus	2%	Watermelons	0%
Groundnut	9%	Rice	4%	Cassava	2%	Broccoli	3%	Bananas	3%
Dry Beans	15%	Wheat	12%	Yams	4%	Cabbage	3%	Apples	2%
Dry Pea	25%	Barley	17%	Taro	4%	Carrots	3%	Grapes	1%
Chickpea	12%	Sorghum	6%			Celery	2%	Oranges	2%
Cowpea	11%	Millet	9%			Cucumber	1%	Mangos	2%
Broadbean	25%	Oats	11%			Onions	2%	Pineapple	2%
Lentil	11%	Rye	15%			Peppers	2%	Papaya	2%
Pigeon Pea	15%	Triticale	15%			Potato	2%	Apricots	2%
Mung Beans	16%	Buckwheat	10%			Tomato	1%	Blueberries	3%
Mean	**15%**		**11%**		**3%**		**2%**		**2%**

Legumes and whole grains, which are the traditional sources of protein, contain far more fiber than fruits and veggies. However, our entire planet is moving away from these fiber-rich proteins toward meat. Across our planet, an inverse relationship exists between the amount of meat a country consumes and the amount of fiber in their diets.[82] Countries that eat more meat eat lower amounts of fiber than those that consume more plants. In the past few decades, average fiber consumption across the entire world has also been dropping as meat consumption goes up. Costa Rica, once again, provides a good example. From the 1960s to the 2000s, meat consumption increased 40% and milk 22%, but their consumption of legumes decreased 44% and grains fell by 31%. As beans and rice fell out of fashion, this led to a 25% decrease in fiber intake. China, which has 280 times more people, increased intake of meat by 183% and milk a staggering 300%. Legumes dropped 91%, driving a fiber reduction of 18%. Both countries have followed in the footsteps of the United States and are now afflicted with chronic inflammation and Western lifestyle diseases that will hold their people back from thriving, healthy lives.

Diets high in animal proteins that have become fads in recent history, such as the Atkin's, ketogenic, and paleo diets, are absolutely terrible for one's health – the antithesis of eating plant-protein-based diets.[252] Cutting out processed carbohydrates as part of their regime may help with weight loss, but the excessive meat, dairy, and eggs wreak havoc on the circulatory system and drive chronic inflammation. Two times more plaque is found in the arteries of test animals fed a high-protein low-carbohydrate diet than in those that were fed a typical Western diet, a diet that already induces arteriosclerosis on a massive scale in our country.[253] These high animal-protein low-carbohydrate diets prescribed to lose weight are associated with increased risk of cardiovascular disease in people.[254] A healthy weight is a goal we all should strive for, but not if it comes with heart disease. What's the point of losing weight if you are trashing your circulatory system in the process? This is like putting a fresh coat of paint on a house that is riddled with termites – it may look better, but it is going to fall apart and collapse. As we reduce animal-based foods in our diets, the key menu items to replace them with are legumes and whole grains. They are protein- and fiber-rich powerhouses that can be adapted and prepared in an infinite variety of recipes and products, many yet to be imagined by cooks everywhere or developed by entrepreneurs in our hubs of innovation. Bring them on. Eat them. Our inner life, the diverse bacteria that make us whole and healthy, will treat us well if we do.

~ Reintegrate ~

The leading trend in livestock production is intensification through industrial-scale feed-crop farms and confined livestock in high-capacity facilities. CAFOs in industrialized countries are the source of much of the world's beef, poultry, and pork production, and similar systems are being established in developing countries, particularly in Asia, to meet increasing demand.[255] At least 75% of total livestock production growth from the turn of the millennium to 2030 is projected to occur in confined systems.[256] Traditional fibrous feedstocks are in relative decline, and protein-rich feeds, like soy, together with nutritional additives that enhance feed conversion are on the rise.[207] As global livestock production grows and intensifies, it depends less on locally available feed resources but increasingly on feed concentrates that are traded internationally.

The transitions away from extensive grazing systems to more intensive production systems, if looking at bottom-line land-use efficiency, present a potentially attractive opportunity.[257] The land footprint of intensive feed-crop-produced beef can be as low as 1/10th of the area required by pasture-raised beef or even 100 times less than some tropical pasture beef.[240] However, many negative tradeoffs result from CAFOs and the intensive agriculture that supplies the feed. It is highly dependent on non-renewable fossil fuel energy to produce fertilizers and pesticides, operate machinery, and globally distribute, exacerbating climate change. It increases greenhouse gases, soil erosion, pollution of waterways from pesticides, hormones, and pharmaceuticals, and causes health problems among local residents.[258] If we can attain a future where only about 10% of our diets is animal-based and focused more on chicken and pork, intensification is an additional, but not optimal, solution to supply this meat. As a powerful trend in the midst of high global growth, intensification makes it challenging to shift to other systems that have lower environmental impacts. By externalizing costs, intensive meat production is making huge profits, and profits mean power. However, better alternative solutions exist. If they can outcompete CAFOs in our market, they can thrive. That will be up to your demand. Your purchases. The customer makes the ultimate choice.

With the release of arable lands that would occur with reduction of meat consumption and replacement of ruminants, an opportunity exists to reintegrate livestock production into agricultural systems that are designed around the structure and processes of natural ecosystems. Smaller, localized farms that are a mixture of human food crops as well as livestock, modeled around the patterns of nature, are the solution. Much of Asia's traditional agricultural systems have operated in this fashion for thousands of years, and this agricultural philosophy is the basis of modern permaculture and agroecology. Ecologically based agricultural systems have been developed by an estimated three-quarters of the 1.5 billion smallholders. These family farmers and indigenous people live on 350 million small farms and put out at least half of the global food for domestic consumption.[259]

In contrast to modern intensive livestock production, within a permaculture or agroecological system, livestock are integrated into a designed and diverse ecosystem that strives to maximize production of foods from solar (not fossil fuel) energy, conserve nutrients and water, and produce little waste. Livestock are not caged as in a CAFO but instead integrated as herbivores or omnivores would be in a natural ecosystem, consuming a variety of feeds, and producing nutrient-rich waste that is returned into the system. Grazing ruminants are valuable resources on natural pastures that are not able to grow crops, and can be a valuable part of a well-designed biodiverse production system. Natural pastures should also be allocated to wildlife, not just cattle. Exclusion of livestock from riparian zones and rotational grazing that better emulates the natural migration feeding patterns of wild herbivores can increase plant biodiversity, build soils, sequester carbon, increase soil nitrogen, increase soil water content, and overall increase productivity and sustainability.[260] In addition to providing food for humans, livestock provide many services within the system. For example, in addition to being fed grains, chickens can be utilized in movable zones to prepare fields for planting. This "chicken tractor" produces eggs and meat, turns the surface of the soil, removes insects and other pests, and deposits nutrients. Pigs can also be utilized as tractors.

Though many permaculture and agroecological technologies are typically used on smallholder systems, ecological designs can be scaled up to operate in larger commercial systems that may produce a variety of livestock, but also crops for local, regional, or national markets. The farmer is not reliant on just one or two crops for survival, but a diverse mix that can not only better adapt to market swings but also climate variability, which is expected to increase. A focus of permaculture is the onsite slowing, retention, and infiltration of water as well as building up healthy, organic soils full of worms and beneficial insects. Earthworm biomass in fields using chemical-based agricultural practices, methods that supply most of our food, have been

shown to be 50 to 100% lower compared to organic fertilizing.
[261] The lowly earthworm is a natural and hardworking solution
for restoring degraded soils as their burrowing and cycling of
plant material gives rise to rich organic, biodiverse soil that stores
40% more moisture and can increase crop yields by 25%. Water,
soil, and biodiversity give us life. We have been mining and
wasting all three of these with conventional farming. With
investment in R&D, current smaller permaculture designs can be
tested on larger areas, learning from multiple sites, while they
become commercial suppliers of products. Better product mixes
and systems will thrive. Poor ones will adapt or disappear.
Markets will decide. Some farmers are trying, but we are in very
early stages. Chickens and turkeys have been integrated in this
fashion into large areas of pasture. After cattle have finished
grazing and been moved to another location, the birds are
directed into the grazed pasture to feed on insects and worms
uncovered by grazing and attracted to the manure.[262] Chickens
and worms can also feed on compost piles. Nothing is wasted.

As in a natural ecosystem, each component of a permaculture
system is linked to many others – relying on many components
and providing benefits to many others. A complex web of
interactions maximizes use of renewable energy and nutrients.
Permaculture systems are designed to best fit into local
ecological limitations and opportunities, and appropriate
products can be produced to supply market demands – local and
national. This is food as we *imagine* it – animals outdoors grazing
in verdant fields among scattered forests, surrounded by
fluttering butterflies, alongside shady clear streams filled with
silvery fish. It is the opposite of reality – confinement of millions
of animals crammed in stainless steel cages, cut off from sunlight
and soil, fed antibiotics and soy from the razed Amazon, whose
shit is sprayed in giant sprinkler arcs of wretched-smelling brown
liquid onto nutrient-saturated fields, poisoning low-income
households and feeding downstream toxic algae blooms that
make water so dangerous your pets can die from seizures if they
drink it. Right now, as customers, this is what most of you are
choosing to eat.

The closed-system, diverse, coupled designs of permaculture systems are reflected in traditional integrated agriculture-aquaculture systems of Asia, which supply diets based primarily on consumption of fruits, vegetables, and whole grains with small amounts of animal products.[35] These systems are based on multiple synergies in which outputs from sub-systems become inputs to other sub-systems instead of being wasted. One species' waste is another's nutrients. The flow and reuse of energy and nutrients between enterprises produces higher-efficiency outputs while reducing external energy or nutrient inputs. Many types of these systems exist such as the rice-aquaculture systems from which fish, freshwater prawns and crabs, snails, mussels, and frogs are harvested, and which may be fertilized with agricultural, livestock, or even human waste sources. For example, in the Mekong Delta of Vietnam, fruit orchards are built upon berms dug from adjacent canals that provide fish habitat and connect to nearby rice fields. Fish and freshwater prawns can move between the canals and rice fields, benefitting from the decomposing rice straw as well as fruit and insects dropping into the water from the trees.

Fish are very efficient at converting food to flesh, and by maximizing the use and cycling of energy and nutrients, these systems can have very high productivities. The area required to produce 1 kg of fish is as small as 1-2 m^2, which is much less than area required to produce beef (68 m^2), pork (19 m^2), chicken (7m^2), or even soybeans (4 m^2).[221] Aquaculture in general can be very efficient at making food and provides over 40% of global aquatic animal food for human consumption.[263] Unfortunately, common modern aquaculture practices that supply developed countries with food, like many salmon farms, are not optimal as they are modeled after CAFOs for terrestrial livestock. They use wild-caught fish for feed, require antibiotics to combat disease in high fish densities, and also produce concentrated waste. They would be greatly improved with more ecologically sound practices based on more diverse species interactions in which the byproducts (wastes) from one species are recycled to become inputs (fertilizers, food, and energy) for another. As on land, these are more ecologically efficient and less polluting.[264] For example, a marine fish farm contained in floating cages produces waste that can be converted to sea cucumbers living below the cages, and shellfish and kelp living down current, all of which can be sold in markets. The fish waste becomes an income source as it is intercepted by other organisms, not only cleaning the water but enhancing economic resiliency. Recent advancements of making feed from algae for aquaculture instead of using wild-caught fish as the feed source is a very promising technology that could help relieve overfishing pressures on multiple trophic levels.[265]

Agroecological systems can be designed to produce a variety of products that are desired by local societies or potentially traded on international markets. Shifting to the kind of integrated system usually employed in agroecology can increase yields by an average of 20% to 60% over monocrop systems, because polycultures reduce losses due to weeds, insects, and diseases, and make a more efficient use of the available resources of water, light, and nutrients. Overall, ecologically integrated farms are more productive than large farms if total output is considered rather than yield from a single crop. We can make more food by producing a diverse mix from a farm as opposed to just growing one item. In addition, these systems provide a much greater level of resilience to climatic instability.[266] However, expanding or scaling up permaculture or agroecological systems has been difficult for a number of reasons, including a lack of access to local and regional markets, lack of land tenure, and limited to no government support such as credit, seeds, or dissemination of agroecological technologies by government extension agents. An underlying and very powerful obstacle to the spread of permaculture and agroecological technologies has been the economic and institutional interests backing conventional agro-industrial approaches, which have enormous lobbying, marketing, and legal power. Research and development for agroecology and sustainable approaches has in most countries been largely ignored or ostracized.[267]

Imagine if we could create rich biodiverse food systems emulating the vibrancy and production of our richest ecosystems – coral reefs, wetlands, forests – that provide us with many hundreds of types of delicious grains, legumes, fruits, vegetables, roots, mushrooms, livestock, fish, and shellfish. Imagine these systems use no toxic chemicals or fertilizers. No hormones or antibiotics. Imagine they are regenerative – building deep rich soils, locking away carbon and soaking water in deep for dryer times. Imagine our streams, rivers, and lakes running clear, teeming with wildlife and splashing children playing with their pets, tails wagging. It is possible.

In the end, it is market demand that will drive a shift toward agricultural systems that are diverse, dynamic, and based firmly in the efficient systems nature employs. Instead of one single crop covering thousands of acres and managed by automated machinery and chemicals, a farm could produce dozens of products, closer to your home so you can enjoy them fresh and nutritious from bountiful, healthy soils and nearby waters. Some crops that cannot be grown locally could still be sourced from national or global supply chains that operate on similar permaculture principles. These systems would be overwhelmingly organic, closed loops, driven primarily by the sun and regenerating soil and water – the base of our food chain. The food may cost just slightly more, but in the long run we save by preventing all those externalized health and environmental costs. We don't need to use massive amounts of fossil fuels, pesticides, or generate extensive pollution to feed ourselves, including the enjoyment of meat. We need to better emulate the wisdom of nature, perfected through millions of years of evolution, symbioses, and biodiversity. We can enhance and harness it with human ingenuity and entrepreneurial spirit. Developing, researching, and managing these systems could provide investment and job opportunities for millions of people to work under enjoyable, rewarding conditions.

Thankfully, these kind of smallholder farms with more ecological principles are sprouting. One of the largest surveys of sustainable agricultural practices and technologies in developing countries examined hundreds of projects in Latin America, Asia, and Africa, in which 9 million farmers have adopted more sustainable practices and technologies on 29 million hectares. Beneficial practices and technologies that were shown to increase average food yields by 93% include increased water use efficiency, improvements to soil health and fertility, and pest control with minimal or zero pesticide use.[268] Purchasing from local farmers is key to supporting this movement, whether you are an individual buying from a local farmer's market or a restaurant fostering farm-to-table. Find local sources and buy from them. Or maybe start your own farm, restaurant, or fast-food chain that can drive supply and demand for people who want to eat for life. Delicious food with a good mission will sell. We all want to do well. It goes hand in hand with doing good.

Chapter 11: **What Should I Eat?**

Of all the rescues that my brother's air ambulance helicopter company has been called on, one stands out as a stark, horrible warning of what not to eat. Brett was not on the flight, but the mission was one that resonated out with a shudder among all the flight teams. On land where the buffalo used to roam by the millions, the helicopter landed out in a field in Greeley, Colorado. The patient was close by but could not be seen. He had died shortly before in a death that trumps anything we could have dreamed up as kids. He was a low-wage worker in a cattle feedlot, in a region where millions of livestock are raised in crowded filthy conditions on corn, soy, and antibiotics, and then slaughtered in assembly lines that turn those carcasses into our burgers and steaks. Trimmings, cartilage, organs, and other body parts are rendered – ground and cooked into a multi-tissue gruel – that is dried and fed to our pets and other livestock. The waste from all those cattle is shunted and stored in giant open depressions of urine and liquefied feces. Literal lakes of shit. The unfortunate worker was driving a forklift along the perimeter of one of these, when he veered too close to the edge. The forklift toppled in, him with it. Morbidly obese, he was unable to escape from its confines. Pinned to the bottom by the machine, alone and panicking in utter darkness, he drowned. His lungs were filled with a slurry of cow shit below that wretched, dark surface. His family was undoubtedly devastated, and I wince with horror and sadness when I think of that last moment of his life on Earth. It is a terrible, magnified reflection of what we are all doing to ourselves on a grand scale. As a species, we are engorging ourselves on animal products and junk food, and surrounding ourselves with the disease, death, and devastation that radiates outward from them. Eventually it comes back to affect our own life.

No one wants such darkness. We all want to feel good. We want happiness. We want love. Being healthy, having healthy loved ones, and living on a healthy planet – these will make you feel better. The most simple and powerful decision we can make to nurture this trio of positivity is what we put in our mouths. Healthy changes in your diet will be delicious, rewarding, and fun. The many negative consequences from our poor diets that I presented in this book – skyrocketing obesity, heart disease, soil erosion, pollution, biodiversity loss – are not the real forces that will drive you or anyone else to change. Fear and negativity are not sustainable motivators. After the near-death terror of a heart attack, most patients will listen to their doctor's ominous warnings and change their diets to be healthier, but typically only for very short periods of time. After four to six weeks, they usually slip back into eating most of the same things that nearly killed them. It's familiar. Comfortable. Convenient. Tasty. New foods can be daunting, hard to understand, and challenging to master after a life of meat, potatoes, soda, and milk. But trust me, there are healthy options out there that taste amazing. I have fed plant-based meals to many a meat lover with rarely a complaint. I have enjoyed a small slice of meat from them once in a while with equal thanks. The joy of plant-based foods, sharing them with love for people and planet, is the best motivator. Make people feel good. Make them lick their lips and rub their bellies with satisfaction. Taste matters most. As with any new endeavor, it will take a little time to learn and be successful. A few bumps along the way with new dishes that don't satisfy you or your family is not a steep price to pay. Don't give up. Enjoy the journey. It gets better and better.

People need love and support, and a sense of community, in order to eat for their life and our life. They also may need some guidance on what to eat. What does a 90P diet look like on your plate? What should you serve yourself or your loved ones? People often ask me what I eat, and perhaps sharing my strategy will be helpful. Maximizing the amount of plant-based whole foods in your diet is the key to healthier people and planet. If you want to reduce your risk of cardiovascular disease, diabetes, and other diet-related ailments while also reducing your environmental impact, you just need to shift the way your plate looks. If you piled up your food from your day or week, I recommend it be roughly divided like this:

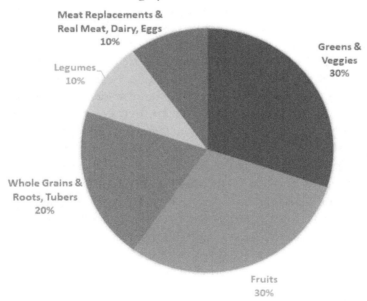

You can also look at these percentages through the lens of total bites of food per day. Researchers have found that the optimal number of bites a day for weight loss and health is about 100 bites per day.[269] I strive first to make sure I eat a hearty amount of greens per day, making up about 30% of what I eat.

Their vitamins, minerals, and antioxidants cannot be understated. As evidenced by silverback gorillas that develop the strength of 20 adult humans by eating mostly greens, the power of veggies is also key to great human strength and health. About one-third of what I eat are mixed salads, kale, spinach, asparagus, broccoli, peas, sprouts, and other green foods along with many other colorful veggies – both raw and cooked. A rainbow painted on a green canvas that can be accomplished through endless recipes, salads being quick and easy. A good diverse salad takes only 10-15 minutes to make and is simple to pack for the day or to make enough to last more than one meal. Many salads taste even better basting in dressing until the next day. Mixing in plant-based proteins gives density and satiety. When out and about for lunch, salads are always easy to find on menus and tailor to your needs – order it without the ubiquitous chicken, cheese, or creamy dressing. However, salads are not the limit. Thousands of delicious combinations of veggies can be achieved in recipes that are warm and hearty.

Our closest relative among all Earth's species, the chimpanzee, thrives on a 97% plant-based diet, with most of their food coming from fruit. Pound for pound, an adult chimp is 50% stronger than a human. Plants fuel strength, and fruits are loaded with powerful and beneficial nutrients. About another third of my diet comes from a vast spectrum of fruits. Every day I start with a 100% fruit smoothie, usually with six to 10 different kinds of fresh and frozen fruit and only water to blend it. Fresh bananas and frozen pineapple, mango, peaches, strawberries, blueberries, grapes, blackberries, raspberries, papaya, and passion fruit. It takes less than five minutes to make, and I often blend in flax seeds, hemp powder, chia seeds, and spirulina. I usually make an extra smoothie, put it in the fridge or an insulated to-go cup, and have it later in the day when I get hungry. Fruit is a staple – the best option – as a snack when hungry, often balanced with a handful of nuts that quickly and easily can carry you through an afternoon. I usually toss a banana, apples, or an orange in my bag for the day out as a backup for the munchies. At night, I may use my Yonanas to make fruit ice cream for dessert, sometimes mixing in peanut butter drizzled with melted dark chocolate.

About 20% of my diet comes from the carbohydrate fuel of whole grains, which are energy, protein, and fiber powerhouses. Part of this 20% sometimes includes roots and tubers like potatoes and sweet potatoes. I mainly eat only whole-grain bread or pasta, but that is not always possible when dining out. Plain white bread or white rice are relatively empty calories compared to whole grain versions, but I don't punish myself for reveling in a great Italian pasta or pizza when dining out if it is not whole grain. Occasional treats are fine. But if I have the option, brown rice is chosen over white in stir fries, burritos, sushi, and poke bowls. Whole grain bread is chosen over white in every occasion feasible, especially at home. The whole grain versions are heartier, more filling, and still packed with protein and that critical fiber that is stripped out from the white versions. These carbs are your fuel – they burn long and strong. Quinoa is quick and delicious hot and cold, flavored endless ways with spices and veggies, with leftovers often mixed cold into a salad.

Protein and fiber from legumes are a must on a daily basis, and I try to make sure at least 10% of my food on average comes from them, if not more, and balance that with a maximum of 10% of my diet from meat replacements or real meats to get solid protein just from plants. A toasted sandwich with a thick smear of peanut butter and honey on whole wheat toast or a tofu scramble for breakfast. Salads topped with tofu, garbanzo beans, black beans, edamame, or chopped nuts for lunch. A veggie burger and wedge fries, curried lentils and sweet potatoes, tofu and veggie pad thai, or whole-grain spaghetti with ground Beyond Meat and tomato sauce for dinner. I have regular items I love, but try to experiment with something new a couple times a week. Keep it fresh. Try something new. Make it exciting. Go on a culinary adventure.

Once a week or two at most, I might celebrate with some eggs, a small piece of high-quality meat or fish, or a few slices of amazing, flavorful cheese like manchego or parmesan. I revel in the experience. I look forward to it. However, I often go weeks or months without eating any animal products, but eventually I enjoy a meat treat while on vacation, when invited to dinner at a friend's house, or at a favorite restaurant. I never feel guilty. Anticipation brings a pleasure that only can be experienced when things are enjoyed as an indulgence, a celebration. Meat never tastes better. When I do eat it, meat covers only a small portion of my plate. I know my body and my gut microbiome is thriving on plants and the occasional treats are little harm, but instead are a celebration of life and its more decadent pleasures. I feast. But only gluttons feast every day. On average over a year, well over 95% of my diet comes from plants – the most important and solid A+ grade I have ever achieved in my life. But that small percentage from animals is savored.

As important as the plant-based foundation of my health, I don't drink soda or any sweetened beverages and I very rarely eat processed junk food other than occasional potato chips as a treat to go with a sandwich. A small splash of olive oil may go into a dressing or to sometimes brown something in a pan. Eighty percent of the items in a supermarket – the packages with added sugar and long lists of unpronounceable ingredients – are things I never have to think about. It certainly makes life easier and trips through the grocery store much faster. It is a simple and easy way to lose weight and live healthier.

In order to achieve a 90P balance in your diet, here are 10 suggestions:

1. Make meat a treat! Try to eat only plant-based foods as a staple at home. Celebrate meat, dairy, or eggs as a treat sometimes when you dine out or only when you celebrate special occasions at home or when invited to dinner at a friend's house. Try to go extended periods eating only plants, even weeks or months if you can.

2. Get some plant-based cookbooks, explore recipes online, and experiment. Invite someone to help with cooking. Make it social. Pick something that looks and sounds delicious.

Discover new ingredients and ways to use familiar ones. A few of my favorite go-to secrets, which can be combined in an infinite tapestry of recipes, are:

Start your day with a fruit smoothie. Use only fresh and frozen fruit plus water to blend it. Nothing else.

Eat a salad, with plant products only, for lunch most of the time. The options are endless and quick-serve salad restaurants are spreading everywhere. Eating a salad also helps prevent that post-lunch lethargy that heavier meals often create.

Have an unprocessed plant protein in your meal on a daily basis: my top choices are tofu, tempeh, lentils, garbanzo beans, white beans, black beans, brown rice, quinoa, edamame, or nuts.

Enjoy processed plant proteins as a treat maybe once or twice a week: meat replacements sold by Dr. Praeger, Impossible Foods, Beyond Meat, and Smart Dogs.

Choose "100% whole grain" bread. White bread is empty calories and "multi-grain" often contains refined wheat stripped of its fiber and protein as the first ingredient instead of whole grain. Look for whole wheat or other whole grain as the first ingredient.

Explore vegan toppings: Vegenaise on sandwiches and to make dressings. The "Just Like Parmesan" by Violife is great shredded on lots of items. Chopped nuts make great crunchy toppings. Use small amounts of real cheese to add flavor, if desired, but don't drown your meal with it. Small amounts of tangy, salty hand-shredded parmesan or manchego go a long way.

Nutritional yeast, boiled raw cashews, unfiltered apple cider vinegar, garlic, and salt can be blended to make delicious creamy/cheesy sauces for mac-n-cheese, broccoli, cauliflower, creamy soups, and topping nachos or burritos. Adapt it with other spices.

Nutritional yeast makes a great cheese replacement on pizza. Just sprinkle. Order pizza with only a light sprinkling of cheese, especially flavorful types like parmesan, or no cheese at all.

Coconut milk, onion, garlic, and ginger as a base with most veggies and plant proteins will please most anyone. It's an escape to the tropics.

Umami is a key flavor that helps bring deeper, meatier flavor to plant dishes. It can be achieved with soy sauce, miso, Bragg Liquid Aminos, and mushroom broth with a touch of salt, or fish sauce (non-vegan).

Balance dressings and sauces with tangy (vinegars, citrus), salty/umami (mentioned above), a touch of sweet (honey, maple syrup), and fermented (nutritional yeast, pickles).

3. On average, limit total daily intake of animal products to a maximum about the size of a deck of cards for meats or fish. Or three eggs. Or three slices of cheese. Or 2 cups or milk. Eat only one of all these options per day or balance a double portion one day with another day eating only plants. For beef, try to eat that deck-size at most once a month, preferably less. Use the animal product to enhance flavor, not to fill up. Savor the treat that it is, which tastes better after days of anticipation.

4. Eat at farm-to-table and restaurants that feature vegan options. Explore new cuisines. Indian, Thai, and Vietnamese cuisines have lots of fabulous plant options.

5. When dining out, mix and match appetizers and side dishes in restaurants. They are often the best plant-based options on a menu and together make a great diverse-flavored meal with perhaps one appetizer-sized meat option.

6. Avoid the center aisles of supermarkets and the sugar and other added junk they contain. Pass on the sodas, including diet. It's junk. Even though it may be hard to quit, once soda is out of your life for a while, you will not miss it. Pass on packaged fruit juices, as they are sugar bombs. If a package lists sugar or corn syrup as an ingredient, think twice. Without sugar drowning so much of your food and beverage, your palate will shift, and you will appreciate its absence. Like meat, sweet is far tastier as an occasional treat.

7. Shop at local farmers markets. They have the best produce, are full of interesting people, and tend to care for the land much better.

8. Buy meat from artisanal sources. They are the healthier and tastier alternative to CAFOs and typically treat animals much better.

9. Permaculture your property so you can eat from your own land. It is possible to easily grow most of the food you eat from a typical suburban yard. In some locations, people can successfully grow 90% of the food they eat from 1/10th of an acre around their home.

10. Share with friends. It is deeply satisfying making someone you love smile with surprise from a delicious plant-centered meal. You will make their life better. It will make you both smile with one of the best pleasures in life. Our communal love of food and life.

Few decisions you make in your life can improve your health more, the health of your loved ones more, or the health of our planet more than choosing a diet that is dominated by plant-based whole foods.

EAT MORE PLANTS!

Literature Cited

1. Morens, D. M., et al. (2020). "The origin of COVID-19 and why it matters." *The American journal of tropical medicine and hygiene* 103(3): 955-959; Junejo, Y., et al. (2020). "Novel SARS-CoV-2/COVID-19: Origin, pathogenesis, genes and genetic variations, immune responses and phylogenetic analysis." *Gene reports* 20: 100752; Volpato, G., et al. (2020). Baby pangolins on my plate: possible lessons to learn from the COVID-19 pandemic, Springer.
2. de Siqueira, J. V. V., et al. (2020). "Impact of obesity on hospitalizations and mortality, due to COVID-19: A systematic review." *Obesity research & clinical practice*; Hales, C. M., et al. (2020). "Prevalence of obesity and severe obesity among adults: United States, 2017–2018."
3. Quinn, T. (1989, August 16 1989). "Colombia records world's highest murder rate." UPI. from https://www.upi.com/Archives/1989/08/16/Colombia-records-worlds-highest-murder-rate/3970619243200/.
4. Gibbs, S. (2009). "Mexican 'drug lord' on rich list." BBC News. from http://news.bbc.co.uk/2/hi/americas/7938904.stm.
5. Pollan, M. (2019). *How to change your mind: What the new science of psychedelics teaches us about consciousness, dying, addiction, depression, and transcendence*, Penguin Books.
6. Cortés-Ramos, J. and H. Delgado-Granados (2012). "The recent retreat of Mexican glaciers on Citlaltépetl Volcano detected using ASTER data." *The Cryosphere Discussions* 6(4): 3149-3176.
7. Gintzler, A. (2019). Bike Commuters Are Dying in Record Numbers. Outside; Ingraham, C. (2015). Chart: The animals

that are most likely to kill you this summer. The Washington Post; University of Florida (2020). "International Shark Attack File." from https://www.floridamuseum.ufl.edu/shark-attacks/; National Weather Service (2020). "Lightning Victims." from https://www.weather.gov/safety/lightning-victims.

8. Murphy, S. L., et al. (2018). Mortality in the united states, 2017, U.S. Department of Health and Human Services, Centers for Disease Control and Prevention, National Center for Health Statistics.

9. Kris-Etherton, P. M., et al. (2020). "Barriers, Opportunities, and Challenges in Addressing Disparities in Diet-Related Cardiovascular Disease in the United States." *Journal of the American Heart Association* 9(7): e014433.

10. North American Meat Institute (2020). "The United States Meat Industry at a Glance." from https://www.meatinstitute.org/index.php?ht=d/sp/i/47465/pid/47465.

11. International Dairy Foods Association (2017). "IDFA Quantifies Economic Impact of Dairy – and It's a Powerful Picture." 2020, from https://www.idfa.org/news/idfa-quantifies-economic-impact-of-dairy-and-it-s-a-powerful-picture.

12. United Egg Producers (2020). "Eggs Feed America." from https://eggsfeedamerica.org/.

13. Allied Analytics (2020). Fast Food Market by Type and End User: Global Opportunity Analysis and Industry Forecast, 2020-2027, Allied Analytics LLP.

14. Franchise Help (2020). "Fast Food Industry Analysis 2020 - Cost & Trends." from https://www.franchisehelp.com/industry-reports/fast-food-industry-analysis-2020-cost-trends/.

15. Grandview Research (2018). "U.S. Packaged Food Market Size, Share & Trends Analysis Report, By Product, Competitive Landscape, And Segment Forecasts, 2018 - 2025."

16. Prager, C. (2020). *Sugar Shock: The Hidden Sugar in Your Food and 100+ Smart Swaps to Cut Back*, Hearst Home.

17. USDA (2020). "Food Availability and Consumption." from https://www.ers.usda.gov/data-products/ag-and-food-statistics-charting-the-essentials/food-availability-and-consumption/.

18. Grand View Research (2020). U.S. Soft Drinks Market Size, Share & Trends Analysis Report By Product (Carbonated Drinks, Packaged Water, Iced/RTD Tea Drinks, Fruit Beverages, Energy Drinks) And Segment Forecasts, 2018 - 2025.

19. American Sugar Alliance (2020). "Where is Sugar Produced?". from https://sugaralliance.org/where-is-sugar-produced.

20. Abrams, L. (2012, November 6, 2012). "1 in 3 Men Can't See His Penis." The Atlantic. from https://www.theatlantic.com/health/archive/2012/11/1-in-3-men-cant-see-his-penis/264615/.

21. Centers for Disease Control & Prevention (2020). "About Adult BMI." from https://www.cdc.gov/healthyweight/assessing/bmi/adult_bmi/index.html.

22. Shahbandeh, M. (2020, Oct 5, 2020). "Per capita consumption of dairy products in the U.S. 2000-2019." from https://www.statista.com/statistics/183717/per-capita-consumption-of-dairy-products-in-the-us-since-2000/.

23. Centers for Disease Control & Prevention (2020). "Heart Disease Facts." from https://www.cdc.gov/heartdisease/facts.htm.

24. Feskens, E. J., et al. (2013). "Meat consumption, diabetes, and its complications." *Current diabetes reports* 13(2): 298-306; Barnard, N., et al. (2014). "Meat consumption as a risk factor for type 2 diabetes." *Nutrients* 6(2): 897-910; Schulze, M., et al. (2003). "Processed meat intake and incidence of type 2 diabetes in younger and middle-aged women." *Diabetologia* 46(11): 1465-1473; Tonstad, S., et al. (2009). "Type of vegetarian diet, body weight, and prevalence of type 2 diabetes." *Diabetes care* 32(5): 791-796.

25. Centers for Disease Control & Prevention (2020). "Prediabetes - Your Chance to Prevent Type 2 Diabetes." from https://www.cdc.gov/diabetes/basics/prediabetes.html.

26. Littman, J. (2018, Dec. 17, 2018). "Report: North American pizza market to grow 10% in next 5 years." from https://www.restaurantdive.com/news/report-north-american-pizza-market-to-grow-10-in-next-5-years/544523/.

27. Baertlein, L. and C. Abbott (2011). House protects pizza as a vegetable. Reuters.

28. Hales, C. M., et al. (2017). Prevalence of obesity among adults and youth: United States, 2015–2016.

29. Schulte, E. M., et al. (2015). "Which foods may be addictive? The roles of processing, fat content, and glycemic load." *PloS one* 10(2): e0117959.

30. Barnard, N. D. (2017). *The Cheese Trap: How Breaking a Surprising Addiction Will Help You Lose Weight, Gain Energy, and Get Healthy*, Grand Central Life & Style.

31. Huang, R.-Y., et al. (2016). "Vegetarian diets and weight reduction: a meta-analysis of randomized controlled trials." *Journal of general internal medicine* 31(1): 109-116.

32. Spencer, E., et al. (2003). "Diet and body mass index in 38 000 EPIC-Oxford meat-eaters, fish-eaters, vegetarians and vegans." *International journal of obesity* 27(6): 728-734; Newby, P., et al. (2005). "Risk of overweight and obesity among semivegetarian, lactovegetarian, and vegan women." *The American journal of clinical nutrition* 81(6): 1267-1274.

33. Benjamin, E. J., et al. (2019). "Heart disease and stroke Statistics-2019 update a report from the American Heart Association." *Circulation*.

34. Lyman, H. F. and G. Merzer (2001). *Mad cowboy: Plain truth from the cattle rancher who won't eat meat*, Simon and Schuster.

35. Campbell, T. C. and T. M. Campbell (2007). *The China study: the most comprehensive study of nutrition ever conducted and the startling implications for diet, weight loss and long-term health*, Wakefield Press.

36. Campbell, T. C., et al. (1998). "Diet, lifestyle, and the etiology of coronary artery disease: the Cornell China Study." *The American Journal of Cardiology* 82(10, Supplement 2): 18-21.

37. Esselstyn, C. B. (2007). *Prevent and reverse heart disease: The revolutionary, scientifically proven, nutrition-based cure*, Penguin.

38. Dulaney, J. (2019). "Frustrations of Being a Plant-Based Cardiologist." from https://nutritionstudies.org/frustrations-of-being-a-plant-based-cardiologist/.

39. Sanger-Katz, M. (2019). In the U.S., an angioplasty costs $32,000. Elsewhere? Maybe $6,400. New York Times.

40. Statista (2020). "Cost of a heart bypass in selected countries as of 2019." from https://www.statista.com/statistics/189966/cost-of-a-heart-bypass-in-various-countries/; iData Research (2020). New

Study Shows Approximately 340,000 CABG Procedures Per Year In The United States.

41. Rapp, N. V., Anne. (2017). Here's What Every Organ in the Body Would Cost to Transplant. Fortune.

42. ScienceDaily (2017). "Cardiovascular disease costs will exceed $1 trillion by 2035: Nearly half of Americans will develop pre-existing cardiovascular disease conditions, analysis shows. ." from https://www.sciencedaily.com/releases/2017/02/170214162750.htm.

43. Paavola, A. (2019, May 2, 2019). "10 most prescribed drugs in the US in Q1." from https://www.beckershospitalreview.com/pharmacy/10-most-prescribed-drugs-in-the-u-s-in-q1.html.

44. Fan, P., et al. (2018). "Recent progress and market analysis of anticoagulant drugs." *Journal of thoracic disease* 10(3): 2011.

45. Heithaus, M. R., et al. (2007). "Spatial and temporal variation in shark communities of the lower Florida Keys and evidence for historical population declines." *Canadian Journal of Fisheries and Aquatic Sciences* 64(10): 1302-1313.

46. Baum, J. K. and R. A. Myers (2004). "Shifting baselines and the decline of pelagic sharks in the Gulf of Mexico." *Ecology letters* 7(2): 135-145.

47. Ferretti, F., et al. (2008). "Loss of large predatory sharks from the Mediterranean Sea." *Conservation biology* 22(4): 952-964; Robbins, W. D., et al. (2006). "Ongoing collapse of coral-reef shark populations." *Current Biology* 16(23): 2314-2319; Bradshaw, C. J., et al. (2008). "Decline in whale shark size and abundance at Ningaloo Reef over the past decade: the world's largest fish is getting smaller." *Biological conservation* 141(7): 1894-1905; Dudley, S. F. and C. A. Simpfendorfer (2006). "Population status of 14 shark species caught in the protective gillnets off KwaZulu–Natal beaches, South Africa, 1978–2003." *Marine and freshwater research* 57(2): 225-240; Randhawa, H. S., et al. (2015). "Increasing rate of species discovery in sharks coincides with sharp population declines: implications for biodiversity." *Ecography* 38(1): 96-107.

48. Ripple, W. J., et al. (2014). "Status and ecological effects of the world's largest carnivores." *Science* 343(6167).

49. Roff, G., et al. (2018). "Decline of coastal apex shark populations over the past half century." *Communications biology* 1(1): 1-11.

50. Reuters (2000). Spectacular Billfish Decline Since Hemingway Days. New York Times.

51. Attard, C. R., et al. (2016). "Towards population-level conservation in the critically endangered Antarctic blue whale: the number and distribution of their populations." *Scientific reports* 6: 22291.

52. Ripple, W. J., et al. (2015). "Collapse of the world's largest herbivores." *Science advances* 1(4): e1400103.

53. Mullon, C., et al. (2005). "The dynamics of collapse in world fisheries." *Fish and fisheries* 6(2): 111-120.

54. McClenachan, L. (2009). "Documenting loss of large trophy fish from the Florida Keys with historical photographs." *Conservation biology* 23(3): 636-643.

55. He, F., et al. (2019). "The global decline of freshwater megafauna." *Global Change Biology* 25(11): 3883-3892.

56. Zhang, H., et al. (2020). "Extinction of one of the world's largest freshwater fishes: Lessons for conserving the endangered Yangtze fauna." *Science of The Total Environment* 710: 136242.

57. Gans, J., et al. (2005). "Computational improvements reveal great bacterial diversity and high metal toxicity in soil." *Science* 309(5739): 1387-1390.

58. Suttle, C. A. (2013). "Viruses: unlocking the greatest biodiversity on Earth." *Genome* 56(10): 542-544.

59. Catalogue of Life (2020).

60. Sweetlove, L. (2011). Number of species on Earth tagged at 8.7 million, Nature Publishing Group.

61. International Institute for Species Exploration (2020). "ESF Top 10 New Species." from https://www.esf.edu/species/.

62. Chapman, A. D. (2009). "Numbers of living species in Australia and the world."

63. Ter Steege, H., et al. (2013). "Hyperdominance in the Amazonian tree flora." *Science* 342(6156).

64. Sodhi, N. S., et al. (2009). "Causes and consequences of species extinctions." *The Princeton guide to ecology* 1(1): 514-520.

65. Huggett, R. (2007). *Fundamentals of geomorphology*, Routledge; De Vos, J. M., et al. (2015). "Estimating the normal background rate of species extinction." *Conservation biology* 29(2): 452-462.

66. Pimm, S., et al. (2006). "Human impacts on the rates of recent, present, and future bird extinctions." *Proceedings of the National Academy of Sciences* 103(29): 10941-10946.
67. Duncan, R. P., et al. (2013). "Magnitude and variation of prehistoric bird extinctions in the Pacific." *Proceedings of the National Academy of Sciences* 110(16): 6436-6441.
68. Boyer, A. G. (2008). "Extinction patterns in the avifauna of the Hawaiian islands." *Diversity and Distributions* 14(3): 509-517.
69. IUCN Red List of Threatened Species (2020). from https://www.iucnredlist.org/.
70. Pimm, S. L. and L. N. Joppa (2015). "How many plant species are there, where are they, and at what rate are they going extinct?" *Annals of the Missouri Botanical Garden* 100(3): 170-176.
71. Riegl, B., et al. (2009). "Coral reefs: threats and conservation in an era of global change." *Annals of the New York Academy of Sciences* 1162(1): 136-186.
72. Contreras-Silva, A. I., et al. (2020). "A meta-analysis to assess long-term spatiotemporal changes of benthic coral and macroalgae cover in the Mexican caribbean." *Scientific reports* 10(1): 1-12.
73. NOAA Fisheries (2019, Dec. 9, 2019). "Groundbreaking New Effort Will Restore Coral Reefs in the Florida Keys." from https://www.fisheries.noaa.gov/feature-story/groundbreaking-new-effort-will-restore-coral-reefs-florida-keys.
74. Jones, I. M. and S. Koptur (2017). "Dead land walking: the value of continued conservation efforts in South Florida's imperiled pine rocklands." *Biodiversity and Conservation* 26(14): 3241-3253.
75. Staletovich, J. (2020). The Seagrass Died. That May Have Triggered A Widespread Fish Kill In Biscayne Bay. WLRN.
76. Brock, T. D. (1997). "The value of basic research: discovery of Thermus aquaticus and other extreme thermophiles." *Genetics* 146(4): 1207.
77. Wohlgemuth, R., et al. (2018). "Discovering novel hydrolases from hot environments." *Biotechnology advances* 36(8): 2077-2100.
78. United Nations (2019). "World Population 2019 Wall Chart."

79. Ballestero, J., et al. (2000). *Management, conservation, and sustained use of olive ridley sea turtle eggs (Lepidochelys olivacea) in the Ostional Wildlife Refuge, Costa Rica: an 11 year review*. Eighteenth International Sea Turtle Symposium.

80. Sánchez-Azofeifa, G. A., et al. (2001). "Deforestation in Costa Rica: a quantitative analysis using remote sensing imagery 1." *Biotropica* 33(3): 378-384; Sader, S. A. and A. T. Joyce (1988). "Deforestation rates and trends in Costa Rica, 1940 to 1983." *Biotropica*: 11-19.

81. Jones, C. F. and P. C. Morrison (1952). "Evolution of the banana industry of Costa Rica." *Economic Geography* 28(1): 1-19.

82. Food and Agriculture Organization of the United Nations (2020). "FAOSTAT." from http://faostat.fao.org/default.aspx.

83. United States Department of Agriculture (2020). "Food Data Central." from https://fdc.nal.usda.gov/index.html.

84. Ivanov, D. S., et al. (2010). "Fatty acid composition of various soybean products." *Food and Feed Research* 37(2): 65-70-65-70.

85. Tovar, A., et al. (2020). "Soy Protein Health Benefits Are in Part Dependent of the Gut Microbiota." *Current Developments in Nutrition* 4(Supplement_2): 669-669.

86. Desmawati, D. and D. Sulastri (2019). "Phytoestrogens and their health effect." *Open access Macedonian journal of medical sciences* 7(3): 495; Nogueira-de-Almeida, C. A., et al. (2020). "Impact of soy consumption on human health: integrative review." *Brazilian Journal of Food Technology* 23; Messina, M. (2016). "Soy and health update: evaluation of the clinical and epidemiologic literature." *Nutrients* 8(12): 754; Zaheer, K. and M. Humayoun Akhtar (2017). "An updated review of dietary isoflavones: Nutrition, processing, bioavailability and impacts on human health." *Critical reviews in food science and nutrition* 57(6): 1280-1293.

87. Hases, L., et al. (2020). "High-fat diet and estrogen impacts the colon and its transcriptome in a sex-dependent manner." *Scientific reports* 10(1): 1-13.

88. Hamilton-Reeves, J. M., et al. (2010). "Clinical studies show no effects of soy protein or isoflavones on reproductive hormones in men: results of a meta-analysis." *Fertility and sterility* 94(3): 997-1007.

89. Messina, M. (2010). "Soybean isoflavone exposure does not have feminizing effects on men: a critical examination of the

clinical evidence." *Fertility and sterility* 93(7): 2095-2104; Povey, A. C., et al. (2020). "Phytoestrogen intake and other dietary risk factors for low motile sperm count and poor sperm morphology." *Andrology* 8(6): 1805-1814; Haun, C. T., et al. (2018). "Soy protein supplementation is not androgenic or estrogenic in college-aged men when combined with resistance exercise training." *Scientific reports* 8(1): 1-13; Key, T. J., et al. (2006). "Health effects of vegetarian and vegan diets." *Proceedings of the Nutrition Society* 65(01): 35-41.

90. Stanworth, R. and T. Jones (2009). Testosterone in obesity, metabolic syndrome and type 2 diabetes. *Advances in the Management of Testosterone Deficiency*, Karger Publishers. 37: 74-90.

91. Domínguez-López, I., et al. (2020). "Effects of dietary phytoestrogens on hormones throughout a human lifespan: A review." *Nutrients* 12(8): 2456.

92. Purdy, R. L., Michael (2018). "International Benchmarks for Soybean Production." *farmdoc daily*.

93. Davidson, J. (2019). Costa Rica Powered by Nearly 100% Renewable Energy. EcoWatch.

94. Machovina, B. and K. J. Feeley (2013). "Climate change driven shifts in the extent and location of areas suitable for export banana production." *Ecological Economics* 95: 83-95.

95. Lindeman, R. L. (1942). "The trophic-dynamic aspect of ecology." *Ecology* 23(4): 399-417.

96. Sutherland, M. A. and C. B. Tucker (2011). "The long and short of it: A review of tail docking in farm animals." *Applied Animal Behaviour Science* 135(3): 179-191.

97. Cunningham, D. (1992). "Beak trimming effects on performance, behavior and welfare of chickens: a review." *Journal of Applied Poultry Research* 1(1): 129-134.

98. Levy, S. (2014). Reduced antibiotic use in livestock: how Denmark tackled resistance, NLM-Export.

99. Steinfeld, H., et al. (2006). Livestock's Long Shadow: Environmental Issues and Options. Rome, Food and Agriculture Organization of the United Nations.

100. Almeida, C. A. d., et al. (2016). "High spatial resolution land use and land cover mapping of the Brazilian Legal Amazon in 2008 using Landsat-5/TM and MODIS data." *Acta Amazonica* 46(3): 291-302; Wang, Y., et al. (2020). "Upturn in

secondary forest clearing buffers primary forest loss in the Brazilian Amazon." *Nature Sustainability* 3(4): 290-295.

101. Tico Times (2015). "McTico? How US fast food caters to Costa Rica." Tico Times. from https://ticotimes.net/travel/mctico-how-u-s-fast-food-caters-to-costa-rica.

102. Arias, L. (2017). Number of obese Ticos has almost quadrupled in four decades. Tico Times.

103. Dieleman, J. L., et al. (2020). "US health care spending by payer and health condition, 1996-2016." *Jama* 323(9): 863-884.

104. Shiva, V. (2001). *Stolen harvest: The hijacking of the global food supply*, Zed Books.

105. Malhi, Y., et al. (2016). "Megafauna and ecosystem function from the Pleistocene to the Anthropocene." *Proceedings of the National Academy of Sciences* 113(4): 838-846.

106. Ripple, W. J., et al. (2016). "Bushmeat hunting and extinction risk to the world's mammals." *Royal Society open science* 3(10): 160498.

107. Gardner, C. J., et al. (2019). "Quantifying the impacts of defaunation on natural forest regeneration in a global meta-analysis." *Nature communications* 10(1): 1-7; Redford, K. H. (1992). "The empty forest." *BioScience* 42(6): 412-422.

108. Wilkie, D. S., et al. (2005). "Role of prices and wealth in consumer demand for bushmeat in Gabon, Central Africa." *Conservation biology* 19(1): 268-274.

109. Estes, J. A. and J. F. Palmisano (1974). "Sea otters: their role in structuring nearshore communities." *Science* 185(4156): 1058-1060.

110. Caughlin, T. T., et al. (2015). "Loss of animal seed dispersal increases extinction risk in a tropical tree species due to pervasive negative density dependence across life stages." *Proceedings of the Royal Society B: Biological Sciences* 282(1798): 20142095; Wang, B. C., et al. (2007). "Hunting of mammals reduces seed removal and dispersal of the afrotropical tree Antrocaryon klaineanum (Anacardiaceae)." *Biotropica* 39(3): 340-347.

111. Kunz, T. H., et al. (2011). "Ecosystem services provided by bats." *Europe* 31: 32.

112. Muscarella, R. and T. H. Fleming (2007). "The role of frugivorous bats in tropical forest succession." *Biological reviews* 82(4): 573-590.

113. Bengis, R., et al. (2004). "The role of wildlife in emerging and re-emerging zoonoses." *Revue scientifique et technique-office international des epizooties* 23(2): 497-512.

114. Karesh, W. B. and E. Noble (2009). "The bushmeat trade: increased opportunities for transmission of zoonotic disease." *Mount Sinai Journal of Medicine: A Journal of Translational and Personalized Medicine: A Journal of Translational and Personalized Medicine* 76(5): 429-434.

115. Young, H. S., et al. (2014). "Declines in large wildlife increase landscape-level prevalence of rodent-borne disease in Africa." *Proceedings of the National Academy of Sciences* 111(19): 7036-7041.

116. Arthington, A. H., et al. (2016). "Fish conservation in freshwater and marine realms: status, threats and management." *Aquatic Conservation: Marine and Freshwater Ecosystems* 26(5): 838-857.

117. Pusceddu, A., et al. (2014). "Chronic and intensive bottom trawling impairs deep-sea biodiversity and ecosystem functioning." *Proceedings of the National Academy of Sciences* 111(24): 8861-8866; Hiddink, J. G., et al. (2017). "Global analysis of depletion and recovery of seabed biota after bottom trawling disturbance." *Proceedings of the National Academy of Sciences* 114(31): 8301-8306.

118. Baco, A. R., et al. (2019). "Amid fields of rubble, scars, and lost gear, signs of recovery observed on seamounts on 30-to 40-year time scales." *Science advances* 5(8): eaaw4513.

119. Rousseau, Y., et al. (2019). "Evolution of global marine fishing fleets and the response of fished resources." *Proceedings of the National Academy of Sciences* 116(25): 12238-12243.

120. Fetzel, T., et al. (2017). "Quantification of uncertainties in global grazing systems assessment." *Global Biogeochemical Cycles* 31(7): 1089-1102.

121. Merrill, D. a. L., Lauren (2018). "Here's How America Uses Its Land." from https://www.bloomberg.com/graphics/2018-us-land-use/.

122. Fleischner, T. L. (1994). "Ecological costs of livestock grazing in western North America." *Conservation biology* 8(3): 629-644.

123. Batchelor, J. L., et al. (2015). "Restoration of riparian areas following the removal of cattle in the Northwestern Great Basin." *Environmental Management* 55(4): 930-942.
124. Rousmaniere, N. S. (2000). *Precious heritage: the status of biodiversity in the United States*, Oxford University Press on Demand.
125. Lange, M., et al. (2015). "Plant diversity increases soil microbial activity and soil carbon storage." *Nature communications* 6(1): 1-8.
126. Center for Biological Diversity (2020). "Grazing." 2020, from https://www.biologicaldiversity.org/programs/public_lands/grazing/index.html.
127. Henry, D. O., et al. (2017). "Blame it on the goats? Desertification in the Near East during the Holocene." *The Holocene* 27(5): 625-637.
128. Pearse, C. K. (1971). "Grazing in the Middle East: past, present, and future." *Rangeland Ecology & Management/Journal of Range Management Archives* 24(1): 13-16.
129. Serra, G. (2015). "Over-grazing and desertification in the Syrian steppe are the root causes of war." *The Ecologist*.
130. Selby, J., et al. (2017). "Climate change and the Syrian civil war revisited." *Political Geography* 60: 232-244.
131. Portenga, E. W., et al. (2019). "Erosion rates and sediment flux within the Potomac River basin quantified over millennial timescales using beryllium isotopes." *GSA Bulletin* 131(7-8): 1295-1311.
132. Goodman, S. M. and J. P. Benstead (2005). "Updated estimates of biotic diversity and endemism for Madagascar." *Oryx* 39(1): 73-77.
133. The Numbers (2020). "Box Office History for Madagascar Movies." from https://www.the-numbers.com/movies/franchise/Madagascar.
134. Global Wildlife Conservation (2018). "Breaking: 95 Percent Of World's Lemur Species On Edge Of Extinction." from https://www.globalwildlife.org/press/breaking-95-percent-of-worlds-lemur-species-on-edge-of-extinction/.
135. Maina, J., et al. (2013). "Human deforestation outweighs future climate change impacts of sedimentation on coral reefs." *Nature communications* 4(1): 1-7; Harris, A., et al. (2010). "Demise of Madagascar's once great barrier reef: changes in coral reef conditions over 40 years." *Atoll Research Bulletin*.

136. Albright, R. and S. Cooley (2019). "A review of interventions proposed to abate impacts of ocean acidification on coral reefs." *Regional Studies in Marine Science* 29: 100612.

137. Union of Concerned Scientists (2016). Global Brands' Beef Purchasing Practices Fail to Protect South American Tropical Forests from Destruction; Union of Concerned Scientists (2016). Cattle, Cleared Forests, and Climate Change: Scoring America's Top Brands on Their Deforestation-Free Beef Commitments and Practices; Selby, C. (2018). Better Beef: Can a remade cattle industry save the Amazon rainforest? Scientific American; Wasley, A. H., Alexandra; and Campos, André (2019). Leading burger supplier sourced from Amazon farmer using deforested land. The Guardian; Johnston, I. (2017). What McDonald's doesn't want you to know about its 'British' beef. Independent.

138. Nosowitz, D. (2020). "Brazil Announces That its Beef Will Be Exported to America." Retrieved 9/4/2020, 2020, from https://modernfarmer.com/2020/02/brazil-announces-that-its-beef-will-be-exported-to-america/.

139. Halverson, N. (2020). "In Nicaragua, supplying beef to the U.S. comes at a high human cost." PBS News Hour.

140. World Wildlife Fund (2019). "Cerrado loses one city of London every three months." from https://www.wwf.org.br/?74546/Cerrado-loses-one-city-of-London-every-three-months.

141. Capehart, T. and S. Proper (2019). "Corn is America's Largest Crop in 2019." from https://www.usda.gov/media/blog/2019/07/29/corn-americas-largest-crop-2019.

142. United States Department of Agriculture (2018). "FAQs." from https://www.ers.usda.gov/faqs/.

143. Gray, R. (2019). "Why soil is disappearing from farms." from www.bbc.com/future/bespoke/follow-the-food/why-soil-is-disappearing-from-farms.

144. White, M. J., et al. (2014). "Nutrient delivery from the Mississippi River to the Gulf of Mexico and effects of cropland conservation." *Journal of Soil and Water Conservation* 69(1): 26-40.

145. Leigh, G. (2004). Haber-bosch and other industrial processes. *Catalysts for nitrogen fixation*, Springer: 33-54.

146. Fields, S. (2004). *Global nitrogen: cycling out of control*, National Institue of Environmental Health Sciences.

147. Mordor Intelligence (2020). United States Fertilizer Market - Growth, Trends, and Forecast (2020 - 2025).

148. Burwell, R., et al. (1977). "Nitrogen and phosphorus movement from agricultural watersheds." *Journal of Soil and Water Conservation* 32(5): 226-230.

149. Ames, A., et al. (2019). "Perceptions of Water-related Environmental Concerns in Northwest Ohio One Year after a Lake Erie Harmful Algal Bloom." *Environmental Management* 64(6): 689-700.

150. Wang, M., et al. (2019). "The great Atlantic Sargassum belt." *Science* 365(6448): 83-87; Oviatt, C. A., et al. (2019). "What nutrient sources support anomalous growth and the recent sargassum mass stranding on Caribbean beaches? A review." *Marine pollution bulletin* 145: 517-525.

151. Fernandez-Cornejo, J., Richard Nehring, Craig Osteen, Seth Wechsler, Andrew and a. A. V. Martin (2014). Pesticide Use in U.S. Agriculture: 21 Selected Crops, 1960-2008, U.S. Department of Agriculture, Economic Research Service.

152. Vera, M. S., et al. (2010). "New evidences of Roundup®(glyphosate formulation) impact on the periphyton community and the water quality of freshwater ecosystems." *Ecotoxicology* 19(4): 710-721.

153. Bowatte, G., et al. (2013). "Tadpoles as dengue mosquito (Aedes aegypti) egg predators." *Biological Control* 67(3): 469-474.

154. Florencia, F. M., et al. (2017). "Effects of the herbicide glyphosate on non-target plant native species from Chaco forest (Argentina)." *Ecotoxicology and environmental safety* 144: 360-368; Rodriguez, A. M. and E. J. Jacobo (2013). "Glyphosate effects on seed bank and vegetation composition of temperate grasslands." *Applied Vegetation Science* 16(1): 51-62; Rodriguez, A. M. and E. J. Jacobo (2010). "Glyphosate effects on floristic composition and species diversity in the Flooding Pampa grassland (Argentina)." *Agriculture, ecosystems & environment* 138(3-4): 222-231.

155. Haughton, A. J., et al. (1999). "The effects of different rates of the herbicide glyphosate on spiders in arable field margins." *Journal of Arachnology*: 249-254; Siemann, E., et al. (1998). "Experimental tests of the dependence of arthropod diversity on plant diversity." *The American Naturalist* 152(5): 738-750; Haddad, N. M., et al. (2009). "Plant species loss decreases arthropod diversity and shifts trophic structure." *Ecology letters* 12(10): 1029-1039.

156. Fugère, V., et al. (2020). "Community rescue in experimental phytoplankton communities facing severe herbicide pollution." *Nature Ecology & Evolution* 4(4): 578-588.

157. Isbell, F., et al. (2011). "High plant diversity is needed to maintain ecosystem services." *Nature* 477(7363): 199-202.

158. Hallmann, C. A., et al. (2017). "More than 75 percent decline over 27 years in total flying insect biomass in protected areas." *PloS one* 12(10): e0185809.

159. Rosenberg, K. V., et al. (2019). "Decline of the North American avifauna." *Science* 366(6461): 120-124.

160. Reuters (2019). "Germany to ban use of glyphosate from end of 2023." from https://www.reuters.com/article/us-germany-glyphosate/germany-to-ban-use-of-glyphosate-from-end-of-2023-idUSKCN1VP0TY.

161. Farm and Ranch (2019). "EPA finalizes cleanup plan for Soda Springs phosphate mine." from https://www.postregister.com/farmandranch/eastern_idaho/epa-finalizes-cleanup-plan-for-soda-springs-phosphate-mine/article_b43cfaea-8b99-5dff-93c4-593e7468020b.html.

162. Gable, E. (2011, March 31, 2011). "Phosphate project near Idaho's Blackfoot River moves forward." E&E News. from https://www.eenews.net/stories/1059947146.

163. Fortune (2018). "Fortune 500." from https://fortune.com/fortune500/2018/.

164. Hébert, M. P., et al. (2019). "The overlooked impact of rising glyphosate use on phosphorus loading in agricultural watersheds." *Frontiers in Ecology and the Environment* 17(1): 48-56.

165. Farruggia, F. T., et al. (2016). "Refined ecological risk assessment for atrazine." *US Environmental Protection Agency, Office of Pesticide Programs: Washington, DC.*

166. Gerbens-Leenes, P. W., et al. (2013). "The water footprint of poultry, pork and beef: A comparative study in different countries and production systems." *Water Resources and Industry* 1: 25-36.

167. Ercin, A., et al. (2011). The water footprint of soy milk and soy burger and equivalent animal products. Value of Water Res. Rep. Ser. No. 49, UNESCO-IHE, Delft, the Netherlands; Deoreo, W. (2016). Residential End Uses of Water, Version 2, The Water Research Foundation.

168. Sun, L., et al. (2018). Economic Valuation for Groundwater resource in Southern Ogallala Aquifer.

169. McGuire, V. L. (2012). "Water-level and storage changes in the High Plains aquifer, predevelopment to 2011 and 2009–11."

170. Steward, D. R., et al. (2013). "Tapping unsustainable groundwater stores for agricultural production in the High Plains Aquifer of Kansas, projections to 2110." *Proceedings of the National Academy of Sciences* 110(37): E3477-E3486.

171. Qingbin, W. and Z. Yang (2020). "China's alfalfa market and imports: Development, trends, and potential impacts of the US–China trade dispute and retaliations." *Journal of Integrative Agriculture* 19(4): 1149-1158.

172. Park, A. L., Julia (2014). It Takes HOW Much Water to Make Greek Yogurt?! Mother Jones.

173. Division of Agriculture and Natural Resources (2020). "Irrigating Alfalfa in California with Limited Water Supplies." from http://ucmanagedrought.ucdavis.edu/Agriculture/Crop_Irrigation_Strategies/Alfalfa.

174. Stokstad, E. (2020). Droughts exposed California's thirst for groundwater. Now, the state hopes to refill its aquifers. Science; Johnson, R. C., Betsy (2015). California Agricultural Production and Irrigated Water Use, Congressional Research Service. R44093.

175. Hoover, J. N. (2013). "Can't You Smell That Smell: Clean Air Act Fixes for Factory Farm Air Pollution." *Stan. J. Animal L. & Pol'y* 6: 1.

176. Harter, T., J. H. Viers, D. Liptzin, T. S. Rosenstock, V. B. Jensen, A. D. Hollander, A. McNally, A. M. King, G. Kourakos, E. M. Lopez, N. DeLaMora, A. Fryjoff-Hung, K. N. Dzurella, H. Canada, S. Laybourne, C. McKenney, J.

Darby, and J. F. Quinn (2013). Dairies and other sources of nitrate loading to groundwater., Department of Land, Air, and Water Resources. University of California, Davis.

177. Watch, F. W. (2020). Factory Farm Nation: 2020 Edition.

178. Martin, K. L., et al. (2018). "Terra incognita: The unknown risks to environmental quality posed by the spatial distribution and abundance of concentrated animal feeding operations." *Science of The Total Environment* 642: 887-893.

179. Novak, J., et al. (2000). "Phosphorus movement through a coastal plain soil after a decade of intensive swine manure application." *Journal of environmental quality* 29(4): 1310-1315.

180. Greif, J. (2020). Redefining algal bloom management pathways in North Carolina, Duke University.

181. North Carolina Public Health (2020). "Algal Blooms." from https://epi.dph.ncdhhs.gov/oee/a_z/algal_blooms.html.

182. Hollenbeck, J. E. (2016). "Interaction of the role of concentrated animal feeding operations (CAFOs) in emerging infectious diseases (EIDS)." *Infection, Genetics and Evolution* 38: 44-46.

183. Adeel, M., et al. (2017). "Environmental impact of estrogens on human, animal and plant life: a critical review." *Environment international* 99: 107-119.

184. Gordon and Betty Moore Foundation (2020). "Andes-Amazon Initiative." from https://www.moore.org/initiative-strategy-detail?initiativeId=andes-amazon-initiative.

185. Amazon Conservation Association (2020). "Threats to the Amazon." from https://www.amazonconservation.org/the-challenge/threats/.

186. Minca, C. and M. Linda (2000). "Ecotourism on the edge: the case of Corcovado National Park, Costa Rica." *Forest tourism and recreation. Case studies in environmental management. CABI Publishing, Wallingford, Oxon*: 103-126.

187. Koebnick, C., C. Strassner, I. Hoffmann, C. Leitzmann (1999). "Consequences of a Long-Term Raw Food Diet on Body Weight and Menstruation: Results of a Questionnaire Survey." *Annals of Nutrition and Metabolism* 43: 69-79; Raba, D.-N., et al. (2019). "Pros and Cons of Raw Vegan Diet." *Advanced Research in Life Sciences* 3(1): 46-51.

188. Cunningham, E. (2004). "What is a raw foods diet and are there any risks or benefits associated with it?" *Journal of the American Dietetic Association* 104(10): 1623.
189. Hirsch, T. (2011). "Brazilian Beauty: The Threatened Atlantic Forest." Live Science. from https://www.livescience.com/30366-atlantic-forest-jungle-brazil-ecosystem.html; Lima, R. A., et al. (2020). "The erosion of biodiversity and biomass in the Atlantic Forest biodiversity hotspot." *bioRxiv.*
190. Saiter, F. Z., et al. (2011). "Tree changes in a mature rainforest with high diversity and endemism on the Brazilian coast." *Biodiversity and Conservation* 20(9): 1921-1949; Thomaz, L. and R. Monteiro (1997). "Atlantic Forest floristic composition for the slopes of the Santa Lúcia Biological Station, municipality of Santa Teresa-ES." *Bol Mus Biol Prof Mello Leitao (Nova Série)* 7: 3-48.
191. Guayakí Sustainable Rainforest Products (2019). Global Impact Report 2019.
192. Simmons, R. (2020). Water pumps converted to oxygenate Biscayne Bay after thousands of dead fish found. 7 News WSVN
193. Menifield, C. E., et al. (2008). "Obesity in America." *ABNF Journal* 19(3).
194. Rojas-Downing, M. M., et al. (2017). "Climate change and livestock: Impacts, adaptation, and mitigation." *Climate Risk Management* 16: 145-163.
195. Machovina, B. and K. J. Feeley (2014). "Taking a Bite Out of Biodiversity." *Science* 343(6173): 838; Machovina, B. and K. J. Feeley (2014). "Livestock: limit red meat consumption." *Nature* 508(7495): 186-186; Feeley, K. J. and B. Machovina (2014). "Increasing preference for beef magnifies human impact on world's food web." *Proceedings of the National Academy of Sciences* 111(9): E794-E794; Machovina, B., et al. (2015). "Biodiversity conservation: The key is reducing meat consumption." *Science of The Total Environment* 536: 419-431.
196. Goldewijk, K. K. (2001). "Estimating global land use change over the past 300 years: The HYDE Database." *Global Biogeochemical Cycles* 15(2): 417-433.
197. Ripple, W. J., et al. (2014). "Status and Ecological Effects of the World's Largest Carnivores." *Science* 343(6167); Ripple, W. J.,

et al. (2015). "Collapse of the world's largest herbivores." *Science advances* 1(4); Steinfeld, H., et al. (2006). *Livestock's long shadow: environmental issues and options*, Food & Agriculture Organization of the United Nations.

198. Nepstad, D. C., et al. (2006). "Globalization of the Amazon Soy and Beef Industries: Opportunities for Conservation." *Conservation biology* 20(6): 1595-1603; Nepstad, D. C., et al. (2008). "Interactions among Amazon land use, forests and climate: prospects for a near-term forest tipping point." *Philosophical Transactions of the Royal Society B: Biological Sciences* 363(1498): 1737-1746; Walker, R., et al. (2009). "Ranching and the new global range: Amazônia in the 21st century." *Geoforum* 40(5): 732-745.

199. Kröger, M. (2020). "Deforestation, cattle capitalism and neodevelopmentalism in the Chico Mendes Extractive Reserve, Brazil." *The Journal of Peasant Studies* 47(3): 464-482; Escobar, H. (2020). Deforestation in the Brazilian Amazon is still rising sharply, American Association for the Advancement of Science; Nepstad, D., et al. (2014). "Slowing Amazon deforestation through public policy and interventions in beef and soy supply chains." *Science* 344(6188): 1118-1123; Gibbs, H. K., et al. (2008). "Carbon payback times for crop-based biofuel expansion in the tropics: the effects of changing yield and technology." *Environmental Research Letters* 3(3): 034001; Macedo, M. N., et al. (2012). "Decoupling of deforestation and soy production in the southern Amazon during the late 2000s." *Proceedings of the National Academy of Sciences* 109(4): 1341-1346.

200. Clements, E. A. and B. M. Fernandes (2013). "Land grabbing, agribusiness and the peasantry in Brazil and Mozambique." *Agrarian South: Journal of Political Economy* 2(1): 41-69; Rulli, M. C., et al. (2013). "Global land and water grabbing." *Proceedings of the National Academy of Sciences* 110(3): 892-897.

201. Brashares, J. S., et al. (2004). "Bushmeat hunting, wildlife declines, and fish supply in West Africa." *Science* 306(5699): 1180-1183.

202. Rae, A. N. and T. W. Hertel (2000). "Future developments in global livestock and grains markets: the impacts of livestock productivity convergence in Asia-Pacific." *Australian Journal of Agricultural and Resource Economics* 44(3): 393-422.

203. Sala, O. E., et al. (2000). "Global Biodiversity Scenarios for the Year 2100." *Science* 287(5459): 1770-1774.

204. Tilman, D. and M. Clark (2014). "Global diets link environmental sustainability and human health." *Nature* advance online publication; Sanders, T. (1999). "The nutritional adequacy of plant-based diets." *Proceedings of the Nutrition Society* 58(02): 265-269.

205. Delgado, C. L. (2003). "Rising consumption of meat and milk in developing countries has created a new food revolution." *The Journal of nutrition* 133(11): 3907S-3910S.

206. Edelman, A., et al. (2014). "State of the Tropics 2014 report."; Green, R. E., et al. (2005). "Farming and the Fate of Wild Nature." *Science* 307(5709): 550-555.

207. Steinfeld, H., et al. (2006). "Livestock production systems in developing countries: status, drivers, trends." *Rev. sci. tech. Off. int. Epiz* 25(2): 505-516.

208. Bonhommeau, S., et al. (2013). "Eating up the world's food web and the human trophic level." *Proceedings of the National Academy of Sciences* 110(51): 20617-20620.

209. Keyzer, M. A., et al. (2005). "Diet shifts towards meat and the effects on cereal use: can we feed the animals in 2030?" *Ecological Economics* 55(2): 187-202.

210. Myers, N., et al. (2000). "Biodiversity hotspots for conservation priorities." *Nature* 403(6772): 853-858.

211. Mittermeier, R. A., et al. (1997). *Megadiversity. Earth's biologically wealthiest nations.* CEMEX, Mexico City, Mexico.

212. Liu, J. and J. Diamond (2005). "China's environment in a globalizing world." *Nature* 435(7046): 1179-1186.

213. MacDonald, G. K., et al. (2015). "Rethinking Agricultural Trade Relationships in an Era of Globalization." *BioScience*: biu225.

214. Tilman, D., et al. (2001). "Forecasting Agriculturally Driven Global Environmental Change." *Science* 292(5515): 281-284.

215. Idel, A. and T. Reichert (2012). "Livestock production and food security in a context of climate change, and environmental and health challenges." *Environment Review.*

216. Altieri, M. A. and L. Merrick (1987). "In situ conservation of crop genetic resources through maintenance of traditional farming systems." *Economic Botany* 41(1): 86-96.

217. Bar-On, Y. M., et al. (2018). "The biomass distribution on Earth." *Proceedings of the National Academy of Sciences* 115(25): 6506-6511.

218. Cassidy, E., et al. (2013). "Redefining agricultural yields: from tonnes to people nourished per hectare." *Environmental Research Letters* 8: 8.

219. Pelletier, N. and P. Tyedmers (2010). "Forecasting potential global environmental costs of livestock production 2000–2050." *Proceedings of the National Academy of Sciences* 107(43): 18371-18374.

220. McDougall, J. (2002). "Plant foods have a complete amino acid composition." *Circulation* 105(25): e197-e197.

221. U.S. Department of Agriculture - Agriculture Research Service (2013). "USDA National Nutrient Database for Standard Reference, Release 26. Nutrient Data Laboratory Home Page." from http://www.ars.usda.gov/ba/bhnrc/ndl; Röös, E., et al. (2013). "Can carbon footprint serve as an indicator of the environmental impact of meat production?" *Ecological Indicators* 24(0): 573-581; Masuda, T. and D. Goldsmith (2009). "World Soybean Production: Area Harvested, Yield, and Long-Term Projections." *International Food and Agribusiness Management Review* 12(4); Prein, M. (2002). "Integration of aquaculture into crop–animal systems in Asia." *Agricultural systems* 71(1): 127-146.

222. Nellemann, C. (2009). *The Environmental Food Crisis: The Environment's Role in Averting Future Food Crises: a UNEP Rapid Response Assessment*, UNEP/Earthprint.

223. West, P. C., et al. (2014). "Leverage points for improving global food security and the environment." *Science* 345(6194): 325-328.

224. Young, V. R. and P. L. Pellett (1994). "Plant proteins in relation to human protein and amino acid nutrition." *The American Journal of Clinical Nutrition* 59(5): 1203S-1212S.

225. Bajželj, B., et al. (2014). "Importance of food-demand management for climate mitigation." *Nature Climate Change* 4(10): 924-929.

226. Laurance, W. F., et al. (2014). "The impact of meat consumption on the tropics: reply to Machovina and Feeley." *Trends in ecology & evolution*.

227. Foley, J. A., et al. (2011). "Solutions for a cultivated planet." *Nature* 478(7369): 337-342.

228. U.S. Department of Health and Human Services and U.S. Department of Agriculture (2015). 2015–2020 Dietary Guidelines for Americans. 8th Edition.

229. Pimentel, D. and M. Pimentel (2003). "Sustainability of meat-based and plant-based diets and the environment." *The American journal of clinical nutrition* 78(3): 660S-663S.

230. Worm, B., et al. (2013). "Global catches, exploitation rates, and rebuilding options for sharks." *Marine Policy* 40: 194-204.

231. All Hands Magazine of the U.S. Navy (2020). "Ready for the 21st Century." from https://allhands.navy.mil/Features/Ford/.

232. Fabinyi, M. (2012). "Historical, cultural and social perspectives on luxury seafood consumption in China." *Environmental Conservation* 39(01): 83-92.

233. Denyer, S. (2013). In China, victory for wildlife conservation as citizens persuaded to give up shark fin soup. Washington Post.

234. Vallianos, C., et al. (2018). "Sharks in Crisis: Evidence of Positive Behavioral Change in China as New Threats Emerge." *WildAid, San Francisco.*

235. Miranda, D. d. A. and G. F. de Carvalho-Souza (2016). "Are we eating plastic-ingesting fish?" *Marine pollution bulletin* 103(1-2): 109-114; Markic, A., et al. (2018). "Double trouble in the South Pacific subtropical gyre: Increased plastic ingestion by fish in the oceanic accumulation zone." *Marine pollution bulletin* 136: 547-564.

236. McCarthy, J. a. D., Scott (2020). Nearly One in Four in U.S. Have Cut Back on Eating Meat, Gallup.

237. Londono, E. (2020). Brazil is Famous for Its Meat. But Vegetarianism is Soaring. . New York Times.

238. Hu, F. B., et al. (2011). "Preventing chronic diseases by promoting healthy diet and lifestyle: public policy implications for China." *Obesity Reviews* 12(7): 552-559.

239. Boucher, D. H., et al. (2012). Grade A choice? Solutions for deforestation-free meat. Cambridge, Massachussetts, Union of Concerned Scientists.

240. de Ruiter, H., et al. (2014). "European dietary patterns and their associated land use: Variation between and within countries."

Food Policy 44(0): 158-166; Elferink, E. V. and S. Nonhebel (2007). "Variations in land requirements for meat production." *Journal of Cleaner Production* 15(18): 1778-1786; Smith, P., et al. (2013). "How much land-based greenhouse gas mitigation can be achieved without compromising food security and environmental goals?" *Global Change Biology* 19(8): 2285-2302; Cowan, R. S. (1986). Beef and Dairy Production in the Wet Tropics. Pasture Management for the Wet Tropics of South East Asia Course Manual, 6th FAO Regional Training course: 193-197.

241. Ripple, W. J., et al. (2014). "Ruminants, climate change and climate policy." *Nature Clim. Change* 4(1): 2-5.

242. Raichlen, S. (2020). Charcuterie With All of the Smoke but None of the Meat. New York Times.

243. Bennett, E. L. (2013). *Hunting for sustainability in tropical forests*, Columbia University Press.

244. Impossible Foods (2019). Impact Report 2019.

245. King, D. E., et al. (2012). "Trends in dietary fiber intake in the United States, 1999-2008." *Journal of the Academy of Nutrition and Dietetics* 112(5): 642-648.

246. Abbott, A. (2016). "Scientists bust myth that our bodies have more bacteria than human cells." *Nature* 10; Rosner, J. L. (2014). "Ten times more microbial cells than body cells in humans." *Microbe* 9(2): 47.

247. Stephen, A. M. and J. Cummings (1980). "The microbial contribution to human faecal mass." *Journal of Medical Microbiology* 13(1): 45-56.

248. Iwata, N. G., et al. (2011). "Trans fatty acids induce vascular inflammation and reduce vascular nitric oxide production in endothelial cells." *PloS one* 6(12): e29600; Mozaffarian, D., et al. (2004). "Dietary intake of trans fatty acids and systemic inflammation in women." *The American journal of clinical nutrition* 79(4): 606-612; Defagó, M. D., et al. (2014). "Influence of food patterns on endothelial biomarkers: a systematic review." *The Journal of Clinical Hypertension* 16(12): 907-913; Bendsen, N. T., et al. (2011). "Effect of industrially produced trans fat on markers of systemic inflammation: evidence from a randomized trial in women." *Journal of Lipid Research* 52(10): 1821-1828; Baer, D. J., et al. (2004). "Dietary fatty acids affect plasma markers of inflammation in healthy

men fed controlled diets: a randomized crossover study." *The American journal of clinical nutrition* 79(6): 969-973; Spreadbury, I. (2012). "Comparison with ancestral diets suggests dense acellular carbohydrates promote an inflammatory microbiota, and may be the primary dietary cause of leptin resistance and obesity." *Diabetes, metabolic syndrome and obesity: targets and therapy* 5: 175; López-Alarcón, M., et al. (2014). "Excessive refined carbohydrates and scarce micronutrients intakes increase inflammatory mediators and insulin resistance in prepubertal and pubertal obese children independently of obesity." *Mediators of inflammation* 2014; De Stefanis, D., et al. (2017). "Effects of chronic sugar consumption on lipid accumulation and autophagy in the skeletal muscle." *European journal of nutrition* 56(1): 363-373; Stanhope, K. L. and P. J. Havel (2009). "Fructose consumption: considerations for future research on its effects on adipose distribution, lipid metabolism, and insulin sensitivity in humans." *The Journal of nutrition* 139(6): 1236S-1241S; DiNicolantonio, J. J., et al. (2015). *Added fructose: a principal driver of type 2 diabetes mellitus and its consequences.* Mayo Clinic Proceedings, Elsevier; Bray, G. A., et al. (2004). "Consumption of high-fructose corn syrup in beverages may play a role in the epidemic of obesity." *The American journal of clinical nutrition* 79(4): 537-543; Raatz, S. K., et al. (2015). "Consumption of honey, sucrose, and high-fructose corn syrup produces similar metabolic effects in glucose-tolerant and-intolerant individuals." *The Journal of nutrition* 145(10): 2265-2272; Hammerling, U., et al. (2016). "Consumption of red/processed meat and colorectal carcinoma: possible mechanisms underlying the significant association." *Critical reviews in food science and nutrition* 56(4): 614-634; Samraj, A. N., et al. (2015). "A red meat-derived glycan promotes inflammation and cancer progression." *Proceedings of the National Academy of Sciences* 112(2): 542-547; Ley, S. H., et al. (2014). "Associations between red meat intake and biomarkers of inflammation and glucose metabolism in women." *The American journal of clinical nutrition* 99(2): 352-360; Apan, A., et al. (2004). "Detecting sugarcane 'orange rust'disease using EO-1 Hyperion hyperspectral imagery." *International journal of remote sensing* 25(2): 489-498.

249. Sochocka, M., et al. (2019). "The gut microbiome alterations and inflammation-driven pathogenesis of Alzheimer's disease—a critical review." *Molecular neurobiology* 56(3): 1841-1851; Bull-Larsen, S. and M. H. Mohajeri (2019). "The potential influence of the bacterial microbiome on the development and progression of ADHD." *Nutrients* 11(11): 2805; Smith, L. K. and E. F. Wissel (2019). "Microbes and the mind: How bacteria shape affect, neurological processes, cognition, social relationships, development, and pathology." *Perspectives on Psychological Science* 14(3): 397-418; Wilson, A. S., et al. (2020). "Diet and the human gut microbiome: an international review." *Digestive Diseases and Sciences*: 1-18; Hills, R. D., et al. (2019). "Gut microbiome: profound implications for diet and disease." *Nutrients* 11(7): 1613; Taylor, A. M. and H. D. Holscher (2020). "A review of dietary and microbial connections to depression, anxiety, and stress." *Nutritional neuroscience* 23(3): 237-250.

250. Koeth, R. A., et al. (2013). "Intestinal microbiota metabolism of l-carnitine, a nutrient in red meat, promotes atherosclerosis." *Nat Med* 19(5): 576-585.

251. Sanchez-Rodriguez, E., et al. (2020). "The Gut Microbiota and Its Implication in the Development of Atherosclerosis and Related Cardiovascular Diseases." *Nutrients* 12(3): 605.

252. Chen, Z., et al. (2020). Dietary protein intake and all-cause and cause-specific mortality: results from the Rotterdam Study and a meta-analysis of prospective cohort studies, Springer.

253. Smith, S. R. (2009). "A Look at the Low-Carbohydrate Diet." *New England Journal of Medicine* 361(23): 2286-2288.

254. Lagiou, P., et al. (2012). "Low carbohydrate-high protein diet and incidence of cardiovascular diseases in Swedish women: prospective cohort study." *Bmj* 344; Zhang, X., et al. (2020). "High-protein diets increase cardiovascular risk by activating macrophage mTOR to suppress mitophagy." *Nature Metabolism* 2(1): 110-125.

255. Thornton, P. K. (2010). "Livestock production: recent trends, future prospects." *Philosophical Transactions of the Royal Society B: Biological Sciences* 365(1554): 2853-2867.

256. Bruinsma, J. (2003). *World agriculture: towards 2015/2030. An FAO perspective*, Earthscan Publications Ltd.

257. Havlík, P., et al. (2014). "Climate change mitigation through livestock system transitions." *Proceedings of the National Academy of Sciences*: 201308044.

258. Juska, A. (2010). "'Profits to the Danes, for us—Hog stench?' The campaign against Danish swine CAFOs in rural Lithuania." *Journal of Rural Studies* 26(3): 250-259; Mallin, M. A. and L. B. Cahoon (2003). "Industrialized animal production—a major source of nutrient and microbial pollution to aquatic ecosystems." *Population and Environment* 24(5): 369-385; Golston, L., et al. (2014). *Ammonia and methane emissions from cattle and dairy feedlots in Colorado*. AGU Fall Meeting Abstracts.

259. Hathaway, M. D. (2015). "Agroecology and permaculture: addressing key ecological problems by rethinking and redesigning agricultural systems." *Journal of Environmental Studies and Sciences*: 1-12; Mollison, B. (1988). "Permaculture: a designer's manual." *Permaculture: a designer's manual*; Mollison, B. C. and D. Holmgren (1979). *Permaculture*, Transworld Publishers; Devendra, C. and D. Thomas (2002). "Crop–animal systems in Asia: importance of livestock and characterisation of agro-ecological zones." *Agricultural Systems* 71(1): 5-15; Devendra, C. and D. Thomas (2002). "Smallholder farming systems in Asia." *Agricultural Systems* 71(1): 17-25; Altieri, M. A. and C. Nicholls (2012). Agroecology scaling up for food sovereignty and resiliency. *Sustainable agriculture reviews*, Springer: 1-29.

260. Weber, K. T. and B. S. Gokhale (2011). "Effect of grazing on soil-water content in semiarid rangelands of southeast Idaho." *Journal of Arid Environments* 75(5): 464-470; Ciesiolka, C. A. A., et al. (2008). "Comparing the effects of continuous and time-controlled grazing systems on soil characteristics in Southeast Queensland." *Australian Journal of Soil Research* 46: 348+; Stinner, D. H., et al. (1997). "Biodiversity as an organizing principle in agroecosystem management: Case studies of holistic resource management practitioners in the USA." *Agriculture, ecosystems & environment* 62(2–3): 199-213; Jacobo, E. J., et al. (2006). "Rotational grazing effects on rangeland vegetation at a farm scale." *Rangeland Ecology & Management* 59(3): 249-257.

261. Blakemore, R. and A. Hochkirch (2017). "Restore earthworms to rebuild topsoil." *Nature* 545(7652): 30-30; Blakemore, R. J. (2018). "Critical decline of earthworms from organic origins under intensive, humic SOM-depleting agriculture." *Soil Systems* 2(2): 33.

262. Strom, S. (2013). An Accidental Cattle Ranch Points the Way in Sustainable Farming. New York Times.

263. Bostock, J., et al. (2010). "Aquaculture: global status and trends." *Philosophical Transactions of the Royal Society B: Biological Sciences* 365(1554): 2897-2912.

264. Ridler, N., et al. (2007). "Integrated Multi– Trophic Aquaculture (IMTA): A Potential Strategic Choice for Farmers." *Aquaculture Economics & Management* 11(1): 99-110; Barrington, K., et al. (2009). "Integrated multi-trophic aquaculture (IMTA) in marine temperate waters." *Integrated mariculture: a global review. FAO Fisheries and Aquaculture Technical Paper* 529: 7-46; Naylor, R. L., et al. (2000). "Effect of aquaculture on world fish supplies." *Nature* 405(6790): 1017-1024.

265. Hodar, A., et al. (2020). "Fish meal and fish oil replacement for aqua feed formulation by using alternative sources: a review." *Journal of Experimental Zoology, India* 23(1): 13-21.

266. Altieri, M. A., et al. (2012). "Agroecologically efficient agricultural systems for smallholder farmers: contributions to food sovereignty." *Agronomy for Sustainable Development* 32(1): 1-13.

267. Altieri, M. A. (2002). "Agroecology: the science of natural resource management for poor farmers in marginal environments." *Agriculture, ecosystems & environment* 93(1): 1-24.

268. Pretty, J. N., et al. (2003). "Reducing food poverty by increasing agricultural sustainability in developing countries." *Agriculture, ecosystems & environment* 95(1): 217-234.

269. Reddy, S. (2014). How Many Bites Do You Take a Day? Try for 100. The Wall Street Journal.

Index

About the Author

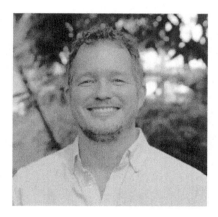

Built upon a lifetime of passion for health and the environment, Brian Machovina is a scientist, inventor, and entrepreneur who has worked for many mission-driven organizations, involving scientific research, teaching, charity, and for-profit businesses. He is CEO of MacEndeavors, Inc., a Miami-based incubator that develops products to improve personal and environmental health. He holds a doctoral degree in Biology from Florida International University where he studied ecological issues related to food security and is a Professor of Conservation Biology.

218